Immune System Control

Colostrum & Lactoferrin

Scientific evidence now verifies what nature has long known - that colostrum & lactoferrin

ACTIVATE REGULATE BALANCE
the immune system!

Beth M. Ley, Ph.D.

Foreword by Raymond Lombardi, D.C., N.D., C.C.N.

BL Publications
Detroit Lakes, MN

BL Publications, Detroit Lakes, MN
1-877-BOOKS11
email: blpub@tekstar.com

Library of Congress Cataloging-in-Publication Data

Ley, Beth M., 1964-
Immune system control: colostrum & lactoferrin: scientific evidence now verifies what nature has long known-that colostrum & lactoferrin activate, regulate, balance, the immune system! / Beth M. Ley; foreword by Raymond Lombardi.-- 1st ed.
p. cm.
Includes bibliographical references and index.
ISBN 1-890766-11-9
1. Lactoferrin--Immunology. 2. Colostrum--Immunology.
I. Title.
QP552.L345 L495 2000
616.07'9--dc21

00-008192

Printed in the United States of America
First edition, April 2000

This book is not intended as medical advice. Its purpose is solely educational. Please consult your healthcare professional for all health problems.

Credits

Cover Design: BL Publications

Art Work: BL Publications and Linda Cole

Research and Technical Assistance: Richard H.Cockrum, D.V.M. and John R. Slama, R.Ph.

Proofreading: Virginia Simpson-Magruder, Jerrita Gronewold

YOU NEED TO KNOW...
THE HEALTH MESSAGE

Do you not know that you are God's temple and that God's Spirit dwells in you? If anyone destroys God's temple, God will destroy him, For God's temple is holy and that temple you are.
1 Corinthians 3:16-17

So, whether you eat or drink, or whatever you do, do all to the glory of God.
1 Corinthians 10:31

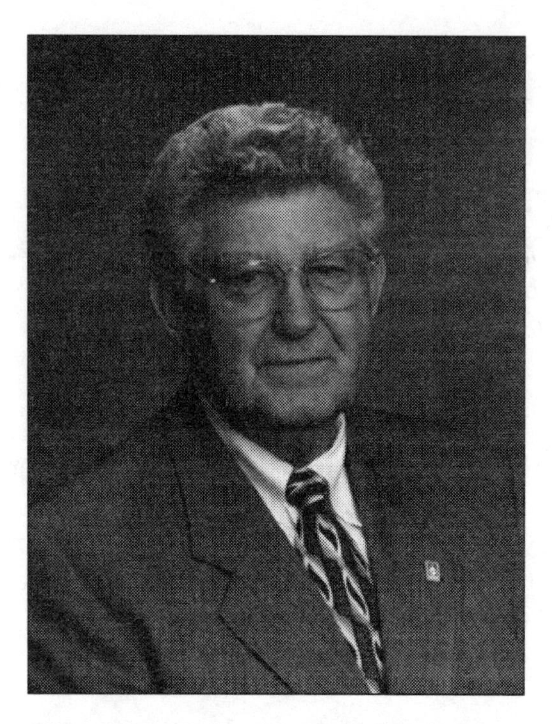

Richard H. Cockrum, D.V.M.
The Father of Colostrum

No man, past or present, has done more for the colostrum industry than Dr. Richard H. Cockrum. His curiosity was peaked as a young veterinary student at Iowa State University when he observed the rapid decline of health and often the death of farm animals deprived of colostrum. Dr. Cockrum's diligent observations of colostrum deprivation in all mammals caused him to start experimenting with various methods of colostrum processing. After decades of work, he successfully achieved a proprietary colostrum processing method that ensures safety and retains efficacy. He has developed a complete line of colostrum based veterinary products that are used worldwide in lieu of antibiotics.

Increasing resistance to antibiotics suggests that it is unwise to introduce one new antibiotic after another. This only leads to more and more multi-resistant strains causing infections that are increasingly difficult to control. It might be better to attempt to reinforce a natural means of resistance, which binds free iron.

C. Gillion Ward, M.D., FACS, J. J. Bullen, Ph.D., MRVCS, and Henry J. Rogers, Ph.D.,
"Iron and Infection: New Developments and their Implications,"
Journal of Trauma, Injury, Infection and Critical Care (1996)

Lactoferrin, an iron-binding protein present in milk (and colostrum) and other exocrine fluids such as saliva, bile and tears, acts as a bacteriostatic agent withholding iron from iron-requiring bacteria.

B. Lonnerdal and S. Iyer,
Department of Nutrition, University of California, Davis

Technology is losing the arms race with evolution. Many scientists believe that the continued widespread use of antibiotics in medicine and agriculture makes increases in resistant microbes inevitable. In the half-century since the development of penicillin, virtually every infectious microbe has developed resistance to one or more of the major classes of antibiotics.

Bruce R. Levin, Ph.D. and M. Lipsitch, Ph.D.,
Department of Biology, Emory University and Department of Epidemiology, Harvard School of Public Health

"Colostrum is an important immunological liquid with proven bacteriostatic and inhibitory activity preventing the penetration of pathogenic microorganisms and absorption of potential allergens into the digestive tract."

Z. Ulcova-Gallova, Ph.D.,
Gynecological-Porodnicka Clinic, LF UK, Plzen.

"I use bovine Colostrum and Lactoferrin in the protocols for numerous conditions. Colostrum shows a broader base and wider application than any other natural substance. I use colostrum and lactoferrin to:

– Retard tumor growth and metastasis.

– Enhance natural "killer-cell" activity (which target specific types of tumors and virus-infected cells).

– Activate neutrophil cells (which surround and digest foreign bodies).

– Prevent bacterial overgrowth in the gut.

– Prevent viruses (including those that cause AIDS, herpes, heart disease, and some types of cancer) from penetrating into healthy cells.

– Reduce inflammation–which can reduce pain and increase mobility.

– Inhibit Candida strains.

– Inhibit free radical production-fighting the aging effects of cellular oxidation."

Kenneth D. Johnson, S.M.D., S.N.D., O.M.D., Ph.D.,
International Orthomolecular Nutritionist

"Most infectious diseases enter the body through or remain localized on mucosal surfaces. What this means is in order to be healthy, we must be able to combat disease-causing organisms where most of them attack us, which is on the mucous membranes of the intestinal tract."

R.H. Weldman, Ph.D.,
West Virginia University School of Medicine and Pharmacy

"The responses have been clinically exciting in my patients using colostrum-lactoferrin lozenges for immune enhancement; especially during the cold and flu season. Lozenges provide protection on the mucosal surfaces of the most where most colds and flu begin."

Raymond M. Lombardi, D.C., N.D., C.C.N.,
Redding, California

"Colostrum is a finely balanced population of proteins produced within the mammary gland. After giving birth, hormonal changes cause the accumulation and production of these finely balanced proteins to cease production. Removal before or after parturition depletes these small balanced proteins and it is replaced with an unbalanced transitional milk which compromises the quality of the colostrum.

After parturition, the mother starts to re-absorb these colostrum components. Research shows that 4 mg. of IgG is re-absorbed back into maternal circulation every hour. This greatly alters this delicately balanced material from its efficacy in regulation of immune responses.

Therefore, only excellent quality colostrum obtained in the first few hours postpartum has the highest concentration of these delicately balanced proteins and is the most desirable for all scientific, animal, and human use. Only a small amount, typically a 125 mg. of excellent quality colostrum in the oral cavity, is required to activate an immune response."

Richard H. Cockrum, D.V.M.,
Perry, Iowa

Table of Contents

FOREWORD

We have entered a new millennium; a time of change, hope and optimism. And we have every reason to be optimistic when it comes to healthcare. As a whole, we are becoming more educated as healthcare consumers, have greater access to information than ever before and are questioning more and more the nature of health and wellness. The concept of achieving and maintaining good health, a state of consistent "wellness," is paramount to a long and happy life. And that is a difficult proposition in our society today, with our fast-paced, stressful lifestyles. Yet, we are learning and doing better in this difficult task. Many of you are integrating better whole food eating habits, exercising more, getting the rest and fluids we need, etc. In addition, there are literally millions of people utilizing "natural approaches" to address their health issues; from taking daily supplements to using alternative healthcare to treat a wide range of conditions and diseases. We have begun an amazing, fundamental shift in our thinking about health and it is leading to important changes in our society; changes that can have a significant positive impact on your health.

As a natural healthcare provider, I am lucky enough to be at the forefront of these changes. In my practice, we see a large variety of conditions and diseases. Because of this, I am constantly seeking natural products and approaches that I can utilize for my patients. As I learn of different products, it is very important to research the various biochemical, pharmacological and clinical aspects of that particular substance. I also investigate harvesting and/or manufacturing techniques, dosage availability and an array of other important information. This is a critical aspect to the delivery of natural-based healthcare within my practice. What this means to my patients is that their protocols are designed around their diagnosis, symptoms and clinical presentation; utilizing the best possible natural substances and approaches that can be found.

One amazing substance that I have had the good fortune to investigate is colostrum. I knew of colostrum from previous coursework while I was in chiropractic college. However, I was not aware of the extent of its attributes and potential usages at that time. Colostrum is produced by female mammary glands before birth and secreted into breast milk. When newborns suckle breast milk, they are getting colostrum as part of the liquid. Colostrum contains a number of important immune factors that are passed on to the newborn through breast-feeding. This is of critical importance to the newborn as their undeveloped systems are at risk for many infectious agents. The secretion of colostrum is short-lived however and has long been considered as something strictly for newborns, not adults.

There are a number of interesting aspects to colostrum, which is produced by the majority of mammals. While I knew that it contained a host of critical immune factors, I was not aware that colostrum from one species (cows) could be utilized by another species (humans). This has critical importance for us as adults, as it has been found that bovine (cow) colostrum can be used by humans; obtaining critical immune factors that we need to maintain a strong immune system. Colostrum, whether human or bovine, contains all four of the major immunoglobulins: IgM, IgG, IgA and secretory IgA. It also contains a number of other immune factors such as leukocytes (white blood cells), accessory factors (immuno-supportive enzymes), lactoferrin (iron-binding protein), polypeptides, etc.

So why is this of any importance? Because we can now, as adults, take colostrum to enhance our immune systems. I have been integrating colostrum into my immune protocols with a variety of different patients in my practice. I can still remember one of the first times I broached the subject with an elderly gentleman with a long history of Rheumatoid Arthritis and immune dysfunction. His response was one that has become commonplace when people first learn that I am putting colostrum into their protocols. He said to me: *"Colostrum? Isn't that the stuff for babies? Where would I get that? Don't women............"* At that point, he broke off and the expression on his face was one of shock. I was quick to assure him that colostrum is available as a supplement and that the form we would be using would be bovine. And of course, that started a completely new round of confusion and questions! While there is humor in this, I consider it critical that the public become educated as to the uses and applications of colostrum for adults.

In my practice, I have approximately 45 people currently using colostrum and lactoferrin in lozenge form. The conditions that I am using it for include Systemic Erythematosus Lupus, Grave's Disease, Rheumatoid Arthritis and Diabetes Mellitus to name a few. The clinical responses have been very interesting. My arthritis patient has noted decreased inflammatory response to his elbows and wrist, with a decrease in swelling and pain. Of the three diabetes patients, all three have noted that their fasting glucose readings have decreased by an average of 10 points. The SLE patient has consistently presented with a lupoid rash over his lower trunk; within two weeks of using colostrum, the rash completely resolved for the first time in 9 months.

The majority of my patients, including myself, are using colostrum strictly for immune enhancement; especially during the cold and flu season. Again, the responses have been clinically exciting. Of the group that we have had taking 3–6 colostrum lozenges a day, only four (of 22) have had a bout of the flu. This may not sound impressive until you realize that the various flu strains have been in epidemic proportions here in Northern California.

Personally, I have been taking a dose of six colostrum lozenges per day for the past four months. I have yet to fall prey to the usual colds, flu's and other various illnesses that typically plague healthcare providers. Please remember that a day doesn't go by when myself and my staff are exposed to a sick patient.

When I was contacted by Beth Ley, Ph.D., to write the foreword for this book, I was both flattered and excited to be a part of such an important subject. This book contains very important information for your health and immune system. I have read many of her previous books and have found the information in an easy-to-read style that has strong clinical and scientific evidence backing it up. This book is no exception. Most importantly, take the information written here and apply it for yourself. Your body and immune system will love you for it.

Raymond M. Lombardi, DC, ND, CCN
Redding, California

INTRODUCTION

People of all ages, nationalities and religion could probably all agree on one basic premise: We do not enjoy being sick. We want to feel good and enjoy life.

Usually we will find that one's health (long-term) is directly proportionate to the amount of time, energy and education that is spent on learning about and achieving health. Long-term, sustained health is contingent upon activating, regulating, balancing and nourishing the immune system on a daily basis. This empowers us to have encounters with deadly microbes and to survive, to engage toxins and to not get cancer, to overcome autoimmune disorders and to live a more fulfilling, healthier life.

The strength of the immune system is directly responsible for our state of health. When the integrity of our immune system is in some way compromised, it is impossible for us to obtain or maintain good health. We must be in control of our immune system. This can be achieved through a daily regime of orally delivered colostrum and orally delivered lactoferrin.

The immune system is activated when it is stimulated. Stimulation can be achieved in a variety of ways from functional foods to dietary supplements. Not all stimulation is good: The immune system of those with allergies is stimulated by an allergen (an otherwise harmless substance like dog hair or grass pollen)–which can create uncomfortable and even dangerous symptoms.

Another case where stimulating the immune system may not be beneficial is in the case of multiple sclerosis or rheumatoid arthritis, where the immune system is already over stimulated. Stimulation, such as the type that may occur with the herb Echinacea, could result in rapid acceleration of the illness. The immune system needs activation without over stimulation.

The immune system must be regulated. Similar to the mechanical regulators widely used on machinery, our bodies need continual regulation for proper function of the immune system. When our bodies become overwhelmed with toxins, pollutants or pathogens the regulatory features of the immune system shuts down. This often results in an immuno-compromised condition. At other times, our immune system becomes over stimulated while trying to combat various pathogens. This can result in an autoimmune disorder. Due to the large amount of these foreign substances and pathogens that we continually ingest, our immune system needs to be continuously regulated.

The immune system must be balanced for the body to achieve homeostasis. Numerous self-help books have been written on achieving balance in life. Our very existence depends upon millions of electrochemical processes that balance the physiological processes that take place in our body every day. Our immune system permeates every aspect of our life and it too must be balanced along with our other metabolic processes. A balanced immune system is essential for long-term, sustained health. We must be in control of our immune system.

The immune system must be nourished. Activation without nourishment is ineffective. Regulation of the immune system cannot be achieved without balance.

Sustained functionality of the immune system must use activation, regulation, balance and nourishment. We have found that the immune system requires specific nourishment to remain an effective force against pathogens and toxins.

I decided to update, expand and rewrite this colostrum book (which first came out in 1989) due to overwhelming and amazing new evidence on certain key elements essential to the immune system. Additionally, new information on lactoferrin and other glyco-proteins is astonishing. This has resulted in greatly expanding and updating this book to encompass these essential elements for the immune system. It is my hope, wish and desire that this book will be instrumental in helping you to achieve long-term, sustained health. This may be accomplished by following a few simple observations and adhering to several long-standing principals.

For this book I was fortunate enough to have two excellent practitioners share their experience in using colostrum and lactoferrin on their patients: Dr. Raymond Lombardi, of the Lombardi Health Center of Redding, California, and Dr. Kenneth Johnson, one of four Registered International Orthomolecular Nutritionists, of San Jose, California. As I was, you are sure to be amazed at how incredibly valuable this gift of nature is, not just to infants, and not just to the immuno-compromised, but to the health of all of us!

"Use food as your medicine and medicine as your food." Hippocrates

HISTORY, HEALTH AND OUR IMMUNE SYSTEM

History of Colostrum

Since the beginning of time, man has observed that newborns fare better, live longer, and have fewer illnesses if they were able to obtain their mother's first milk.

In America, the Amish are claimed to have celebrated the beginning of a new life when a calf was born. After the calf's first feeding, they harvested the colostrum (or first milk) and prepared a pudding from it for the whole family to enjoy. The Amish noted for decades the health benefits of such a ritual. It appears that the ritual was eventually lost or replaced.

In India, where cows are sacred, colostrum is still delivered to the doorstep along with the normal milk delivery. When illness strikes a household, colostrum is often the first medication used by the family.

What Happened to Tradition?

The way we view life and health has changed dramatically over the last hundred years. So have our lifestyles and our morality. In America, and more recently in other parts of the world, we have become a quick-fix, disposable society. Convenience and self-indulgence have become a mainstay of our lives. This phenomenon has permeated every aspect of our lives. Jobs, family, shopping, healthcare; we are continually bombarded with marketing efforts that show us how to obtain something quickly and easily that will enhance our appearance, status, health or wealth.

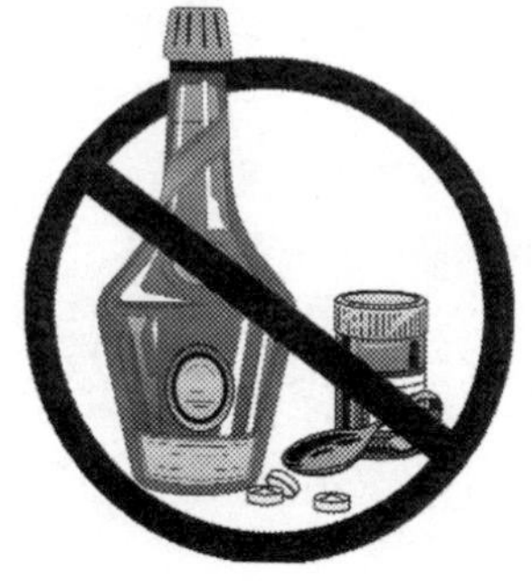

Shortly after the turn of the century, Congress enacted prohibition, which caused the demise of the saloon. This quickly gave rise to the speak-easy, a place to drink in secret. The speak-easy finally evolved to the "club" for drinking, dancing and socializing. This helped to increase acceptance, consumption and addiction to alcohol. Around this same time the cigarette was born, which ushered in a new era for the tobacco industries and increased tobacco addiction ten-fold. Over the course of a few decades, drinking and smoking were no longer a habit restricted to the affluent male.

In financial circles new ideas improved the quality of life and created new stress. Financial ingenuity gave rise to a new product called the mortgage. A new stress appeared on the horizon when we no longer had to save up for a house like our grandparents did. We were able to "buy it now" and pay for later by taking out a mortgage. This philosophy was later expanded to consumer goods with the advent of the credit card. Over-extending ourselves became the American way. The quick-fix for over spending and self-indulgence would be to claim bankruptcy, which in turn created even more stress.

In our youth we thought we were invincible and that no matter what we ate, drank or smoked, no matter what kind of hours we kept or the amount of stress we allowed ourselves to accumulate, we thought that we would stay healthy, full of energy, and feel great forever. Now here we are years later with joint pain, headaches, skin problems, high blood pressure, elevated blood lipids, memory loss, weight problems, irritability, can't stay awake after 10 p.m. and so on. What we realize now is that many of the factors that regulate how we feel are under our control. We can abuse our health and wear it down, making us more susceptible to ill health and premature aging, or we can support it and sustain its ability to protect us for years to come.

As our grandparents and parents become older and die, so do many of the traditions that they passed on through generations. We have often chosen to forsake tradition for convenience and self-indulgence. There may be nothing wrong with an occasional glass of wine or cocktail, having a home mortgage or a credit card balance. The point is that we, as a society, are continually looking for the easy way out and that this quick fix philosophy has resulted in the gradual erosion of tradition.

This philosophy has impacted every facet of our life: Our health, the stress we subject ourselves to, the way we view medicine and the pollution of our environment. Now we face Ebola, West Nile virus and other frightening diseases. These new diseases are occurring at an alarming rate. Pathogens are being observed where previously there were none–superbugs that are unaffected by our current arsenal of antibiotics. Toxins are now commonplace that were unheard of just decades ago. Obesity is at a record high, notwithstanding a myriad of low-fat foods. Even with all the high technology the world has to offer, we have succumbed to a much poorer quality of life than that of previous generations.

Why We Die So Young

Natural human life span is believed to be at least 120 years, yet most of us die prematurely at age 73 for men and at age 77 for women. Why? If we do not provide the body with what it needs to function properly, we cannot adequately fight off illness and disease. Inadequate immune function leaves us vulnerable to recurrent or degenerative conditions or those concentrated in specific organs, such as the lungs, heart or reproductive system. Eventually, cancer, AIDS or some other opportunistic disease takes over.

Good health should not be thought of as the absence of disease. We should avoid this negative disease-orientated thinking and try to concentrate on what we must to do to remain healthy. Health results from supplying what is essential to the body on a daily basis, while disease results from living without what the body needs. We are responsible for our own health and should take control of it. When we are in control of our health, disease can not take over.

It is not normal to be sick all the time. It is normal for the body to continually fight off whatever it encounters. Cancerous cells, for example, are in the body at all times. Normally, cells of the immune system are able to keep them in check so that they do not cause harm. Every day we are faced with infectious and opportunistic organisms ranging from E. coli to

HIV. Under normal conditions, thanks to our immune system, they do not bother us and we do not even know they are present.

But, if the immune system is overworked by fighting off toxins that we continually subject it to, our immune system eventually breaks down. We often voluntarily subject it to toxins from cigarettes, drugs, highly processed foods, unsafe water and polluted air. At other times we involuntarily subject our system to toxins by consuming pesticide-laced foods, by adhering to the routine prescription of antibiotics, and stress imposed by our job, family and even our friends. Eventually we overwhelm our immune system and it breaks down, leaving us vulnerable to numerous illnesses and diseases.

Who is in charge of our health?

Each individual is in charge of their health. Our health is supported by new, creative developments in the healthcare industry; however, we are currently feeling the effects of our poor decisions in the management of new technology over the past five decades.

Our decisions have resulted in:

- New strains of bacteria and viruses that are resistant to existing antibiotics
- Chemical pollutants in our food, water and air resulting in compromised immune systems
- Highly processed nutrient deficient foods resulting in cell and digestive system degradation
- Overwhelmed immune systems due to job and family stresses
- Impaired tissue and muscle repair due to pushing

the body beyond its natural limits and as a natural result of aging

Over-reliance and Misuse of Drugs

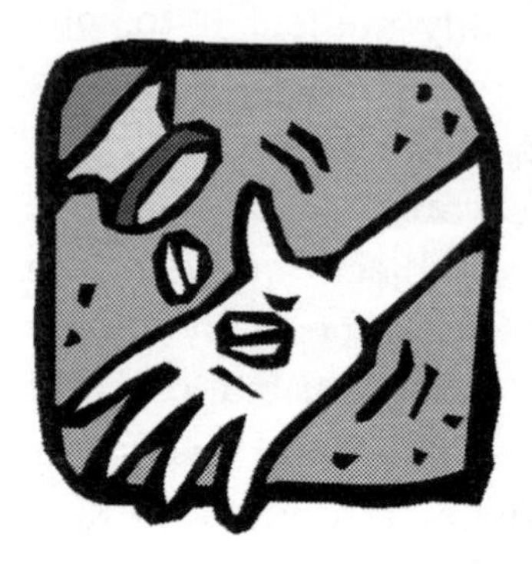

Drugs are not the answer for optimal health, immunity and long lives. In fact, they often create more problems than they help us. Drugs give us quick relief, a bandage to cover up what we do not want to face. Pain and other "symptoms" are signs that something is wrong, that our immune system is unable "to keep up." Instead of taking a look at our diet and lifestyles, we turn to:

- Antihistamines and nasal sprays that mask the symptoms of colds, allergies and sinusitis

- Antibiotics, especially for children who need to develop an immune system on their own, to ward off infections or to clear up acne

- Crash diets or diet pills to help us lose weight

- Caffeine and sweets to give us quick energy

- Alcohol, tranquilizers or valium to relieve stress and help us sleep; or any other quick-fix solutions

Let's take a took at what we should be doing instead.

TAKE CONTROL OF YOUR IMMUNE SYSTEM

A healthy immune system keeps the entire body in a state of balance.

Without optimal immune protection we are susceptible to conditions ranging from the common cold, the flu, various stages of immune deficiency, cancer and even AIDS.

It is the responsibility of the immune system to protect us from these conditions. We may take immunity for granted until we are threatened with losing it. Research now shows that much of the efficiency of the immune system may depend greatly upon ourselves.

The good news is that you can take control. You can restore and revitalize your immune system. You don't have to be prey to catch every cold and virus that comes along, you do not have to experience aches and pains, you do not have to feel stressed all the time. You can rid your body of toxins and chemicals, you can lose that excess weight, you can enjoy restful sleep, and you can improve your memory and concentration. You can enjoy life!

If you want to live your life to the fullest, full of vitality, free of pain and illness, you must simply commit to making a few simple changes. The changes are not easy, but they are simple. Taking control of your immune system, health and life can be accomplished by doing the following:

1. Educate Yourself on Nutrition

While many of us often prefer to eat for the enjoyment of food, the nutrition of the food we eat is critical for our long-term health. Knowledge of the nutrients and their functions in the body is needed for the understanding of how diet influences our health.

Nutrition is the relationship between foods and the health of the body. Optimal nutrition is a diet that contains all essential nutrients which are supplied and utilized in a balanced amount to maintain health.

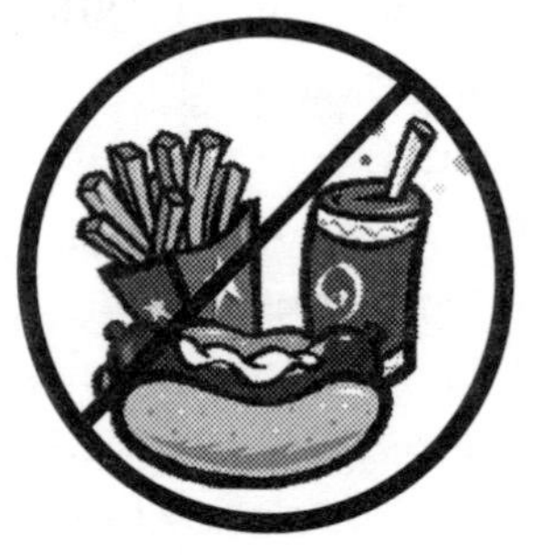

A balanced diet contains proper portions of each of the main nutrient classifications of food: Carbohydrates, proteins, fats, vitamins, minerals and water. Additional components of a healthy diet include enzymes, antioxidants and fiber which have their own important contributions to good health and longevity.

Each nutrient has its own special function and relationship to the body, but no nutrient acts independently of the other nutrients. The body functions best when all the needed nutrients are present in their proper proportions. A shortage of just one can weaken the system.

For a number of reasons, individuals often do not get all they need of certain vitamins and minerals in their diet. Crops are grown in mineral-deficient soil. Synthetic and super-phosphate fertilizers, pesticides, herbicides, growth regulators and livestock feed additives destroy microbial soil life needed to make the soil nutrients available to the plant. Heavy rain and irrigation can even wash away water-soluble nutrients.

Vitamins and minerals play a key role in the effectiveness of the immune system. A Lack of vitamin A lowers the number of T-cells and effects the integrity of the mucous linings. Vitamin B deficiencies, especially B-6 and B-12, decrease our ability to produce germ-fighting antibodies. Vitamin C (which itself is anti-viral) is needed for optimal macrophage activity. Zinc deficiencies cause many of the lymph tissues to shrink. The thymus gland, for example, where T cells develop, and lymph nodes, where white blood cells are stored until needed, are affected. Low zinc levels also reduce macrophage activity and T-cell numbers. Low levels of selenium reduce antibodies.

Amino acids such as tryptophan, phenylalanine, lysine and methionine, are needed in adequate amounts to produce antibodies and also T-cells. In all, there are over 50 different nutrients which are needed for optimal immune function.

Good nutrition is essential for normal organ development and functioning, for normal reproduction, for growth, for optimal energy and efficiency, for resistance to infection and disease, and for the ability to repair bodily damage or injury. It all relates to immunity.

It is our own responsibility to feed ourselves properly. We cannot expect to maintain optimal functioning as a human living machine if we feed it junk - calories devoid of crucial nutrients. As a nation of convenience, we have grown accustomed to what is fast and easy. Frozen, pre-packaged, boxed, quick-cooking and "fast" foods have replaced what once took our grandmothers all day to prepare. These "fast" foods lack vital nutrients, fiber and enzymes, which we truly need for optimal immunity.

Nationwide surveys in North America have shown that the diets of more than 60% of the people tested did not even obtain the very low recommended Daily Values (DV) of all essential nutrients and have one or more deficiencies. The DV are the minimal requirements for these nutrients and are inadequate to maintain optimum health.

The most common deficiencies found in these surveys were vitamins C, A, E, B-6, B-2, folic acid, iron, calcium, zinc, chromium, iodine, magnesium, selenium, manganese and essential fatty acids.

Deficiency symptoms are not necessarily obvious. Conditions develop slowly over time. One does not need to have scurvy to have a vitamin C deficiency or osteoporosis to have a calcium deficiency. Symptoms can be as subtle as appetite loss, bad breath, soft or brittle fingernails, fatigue or insomnia.

While we suffer from colds, sinusitis, allergies, excessive weight, diabetes, hypoglycemia, anemia, arthritis, mental problems, depression, heart disease, cancer and many other conditions that leave us unsatisfied with our health and feeling rotten, we too often do not even consider our own eating habits as the possible cause.

Concentrate on eating simple, nutritious foods; soups; whole grains; fresh fruits and vegetables and their juices; and lots of liquids (particularly pure water), to help flush toxins, etc. out the body. Avoid processed foods, sugar, caffeine, alcohol and tobacco.

2. Take Time for Yourself to Get Proper Rest and Reduce Stress

Studies have shown that the immune system functions best while we are asleep. Deep sleep is important for immune function, for example, B-cell and macrophage activity increases. The body needs to shut down in order for the immune system to effectively fight off what it has encountered. Most people know that we tend to sleep more when we are sick. Therefore, it seems obvious that we must need it. Lack of sleep, insomnia and irregular sleeping habits (common with irregular work hours) have been shown to be detrimental to health and longevity.

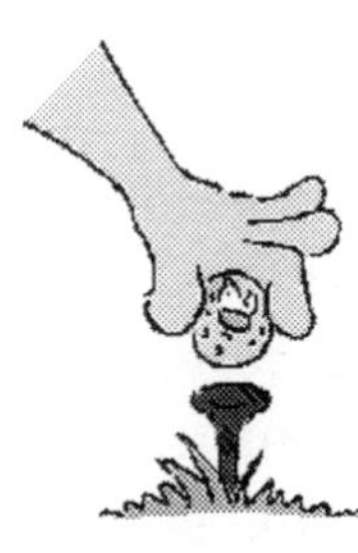

Taking time out on a regular basis to do the things you enjoy–playing golf or tennis, going fishing or bike riding, going to the movies, listening to music, playing chess, reading a good book or simply spending time with friends and family, etc., is an important part of maintaining good health. This is needed to relieve stress, and simply make life more enjoyable.

3. Maintain a Good Attitude

A positive attitude and desire for wellness is always of importance for optimal health. You may have heard the saying "laughter is the best medicine." It may not work alone, but it is a very important component of good health.

4. Maintain Proper Hygiene

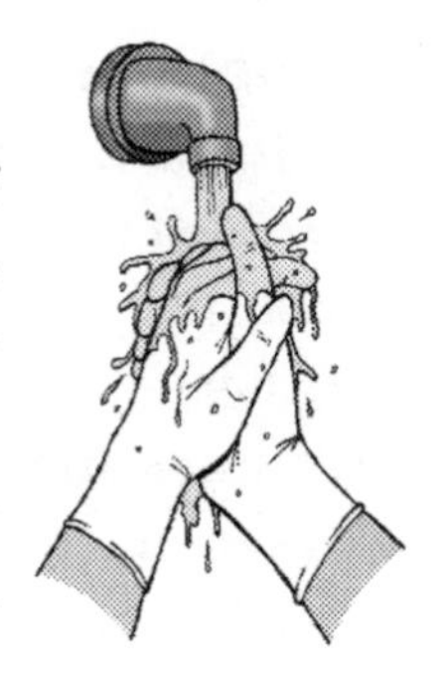

Many infections could be avoided if we would simply wash our hands more often – as often as 10 or 15 times a day if in a high-risk contaminated environments (public bathrooms, office buildings, high-use pay phones, etc.). Avoid touching your face, mouth, eyes, etc. as much as possible. If you know that infected individuals are using the same phone, keyboard, etc., as you it is a good idea to disinfect them or not share even simple objects such as pens.

5. Properly Supplement Your Immune System

Colostrum and lactoferrin activate, regulate and balance the immune system. Nourishment is another issue.

Nutritional Support: Vitamin B Complex, vitamin C, E, zinc, selenium and other nutritional support factors may be critical for speedy recovery.

Dr. Linus Pauling told us the body requires large doses as high as 20-40+ grams of vitamin C per day in times of stress and illness. Vitamin C stimulates the production of interferon and increases the activity of certain white blood cells.

Other nutrients are just as important: Vitamin B-5 is needed to make antibodies and for normal adrenal functioning. Vitamin A can greatly increase the size and effectiveness of the thymus gland. Zinc, containing anti-bacterial/viral properties, is important for the health of the immune system.

Antioxidants: Vitamins A, C and E, beta carotene, bioflavonoids, zinc, selenium, lipoic acid and CoQ10 are extremely important antioxidants which help protect us from the damage of free radicals formed normally in our body and by exposure to pollutants in our air, food and water. It is a good idea to supplement a variety of antioxidants as they individually are less effective compared to when taken collectively. Certain antioxidants are more effective than others against specific types of free radicals.

Herbal Support: There are perhaps hundreds of herbs to strengthen the immune system. The best known of these include Echinacea, Golden Seal, Garlic, Burdock root, Licorice root, Marshmallow and Pau D'Arco.

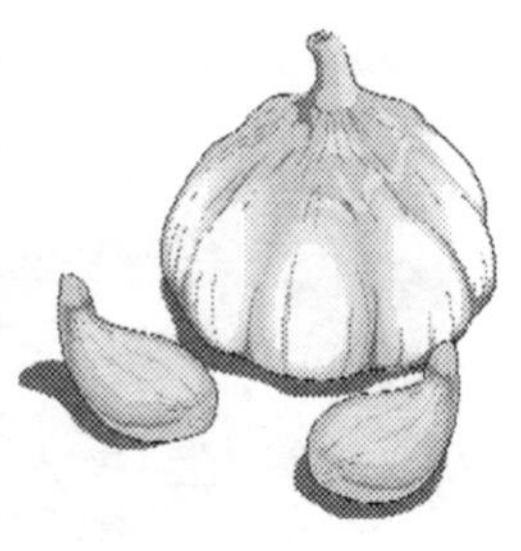

Additional Suggested Supplements:

Essential Fatty Acids (DHA and EPA) such as Evening Primrose Oil, Flax Seed Oil, Fish Oils, etc.

Probiotics (Friendly intestinal bacteria such as L. Acidophilus and Bifidus)

Spirulina (Blue-green algae)

MSM (Rich source of organic sulfur)

You can't just take a pill...

This book is too small to cover in detail all of the components of a healthy immune system and a healthy person's life, i.e. spiritual beliefs, mental health, love, relationships and exercise. However, each one is extremely important for good health.

The naturopathic medicinal approach to health and healing is consistent with the body, working with it rather than against it. This was the philosophy of many traditional remedies which have now been lost or replaced.

Chicken soup was a traditional remedy for illnesses such as cold and flu. Today we know that valuable phytonutrients found in garlic, onion, carrots, etc. all enhance immunity. The heat of the broth also encourages body temperature to raise. Fever is a natural immune response against bacteria and viruses.

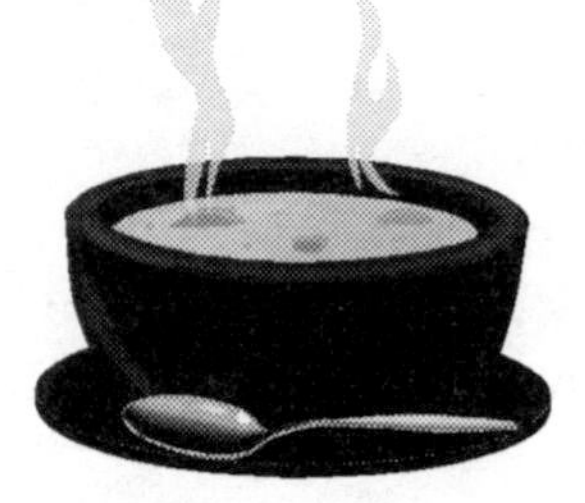

Not all so-called natural remedies are the answer to every ailment. Numerous companies make inappropriate unsubstantiated claims for their products just to increase sales. We need to be able to sort through the mass of information and misinformation to make educated decisions for ourselves.

Take the example of weight loss. It is much more complicated than just taking an herb or vitamin. You cannot just take some magic pill, sit around all day eating ice cream, chips and chocolate and expect to look like Arnold Schwarzenegger, Madonna, Cindy Crawford or whoever represents your ideal male or female body type. Supplements do not work by themselves. There are no miracle cures for weight loss. Diet, exercise and proper nutrition are all essential. Supplements can only help the process.

The natural approach maintains that the constant effort of the body's life force is always in the direction of self-cleansing, self-repairing and positive health. The philosophy maintains that even acute disease is a manifestation of the body's efforts in the direction of self-cure. Disease, or downgraded health, may be eliminated only by removing the real cause from the system and by raising the body's general vitality so that its natural and inherent ability to sustain health is allowed to dominate. In short, this means taking control of your immune system and balancing all body functions.

Natural therapeutic philosophy also maintains that chronic diseases are frequently the result of mistaken efforts to cure or attempted suppression of the physiological efforts of the body to cleanse itself. (Lindlahr)

Thanks to the research stimulated by Dr. Linus Pauling and other nutrition "forefathers," we now realize the astounding health-protective, immune-stimulating factors of vitamin C and other substances found in nature. Recently an increasing amount of scientific attention has also been devoted to other naturally occurring substances. In a sense, we are moving back to basics. The best medicine may have been under our noses the entire time. It is the least expensive – the least drastic – that can gently lead our body back to homeostasis.

More research needs to be done on an endless array of natural compounds to determine their potential to benefit our health, but research is expensive. While pharmaceutical companies fund a large number of health-related research studies, they are not so interested in funding research for natural products, which cannot be patented.

IMMUNITY

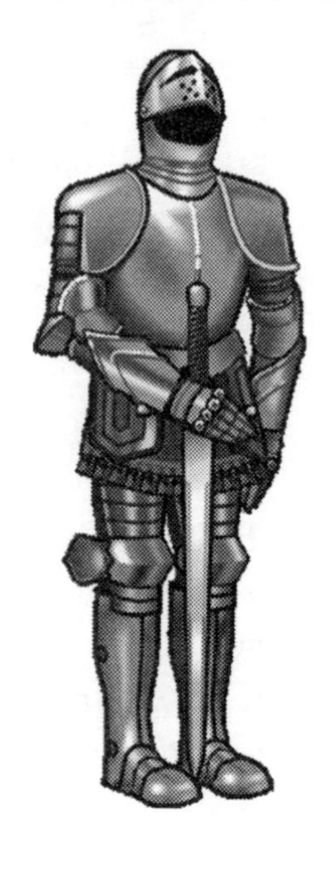

Immunity is the ability of the body to overcome infection, injury and disease-producing organisms, and to recognize certain substances as foreign and to neutralize or eliminate them. The human body continually attempts to maintain homeostasis by counteracting the harmful stimuli it encounters. The immune defenses represent a variety of body reactions including the production of a specific antibody against each stimuli. It combats microbial invasion, provides resistance against the development of communicable and virulent diseases and eliminates undesirable substances from the body.

The immune system is responsible for maintaining homeostasis in every part of the body. It has duties that range from cleaning the lungs of foreign particles we inhale, to searching out and destroying invaders like infectious microorganisms and ridding the body of cancerous cells to affecting our attitudes and our sex drive. The effects of the immune system reach every aspect of our life.

The Root of All Disease: A Faulty Immune System

The importance of the immune system cannot be overstated. The immune system is essential for human survival. It protects us not only from "invaders" such as yeast, bacteria and viruses, but also from substances such as alcohol, tobacco and caffeine. Without a properly functioning immune system, good health cannot be maintained because an individual cannot clean out or destroy the invaders.

The human body continually attempts to maintain homeostasis by counteracting the invaders it encounters. The immune defenses involve a variety of body reactions including the production of a specific antibody against the antigen it encounters. This is known as the antigen-antibody response. Whenever that specific antigen (ragweed pollen, for example) enters the body again, the immune system "remembers" and immediately forms its antibodies against it.

The normal functioning of the immune system is vital for good health and life. "***In the complete absence of the immune function, human survival is not possible for more than a day or so before overwhelming infection leads to death.***" (Snyderman)

How the Immune System Works

The immune system is one of the most complex systems of the body. It is highly interactive with itself and with the other systems of the body. It is impossible to remove or replace the immune system.

The immune system consists of the thymus, thyroid, spleen, bone marrow, adrenal glands, lymphatic vessels, lymph nodes (including the tonsils), specialized white blood cells such as the B-cells, T-cells (killer, helper, and suppressor), macrophage "scavenger" cells, and antibodies. Each has a different responsibility but they all function together.

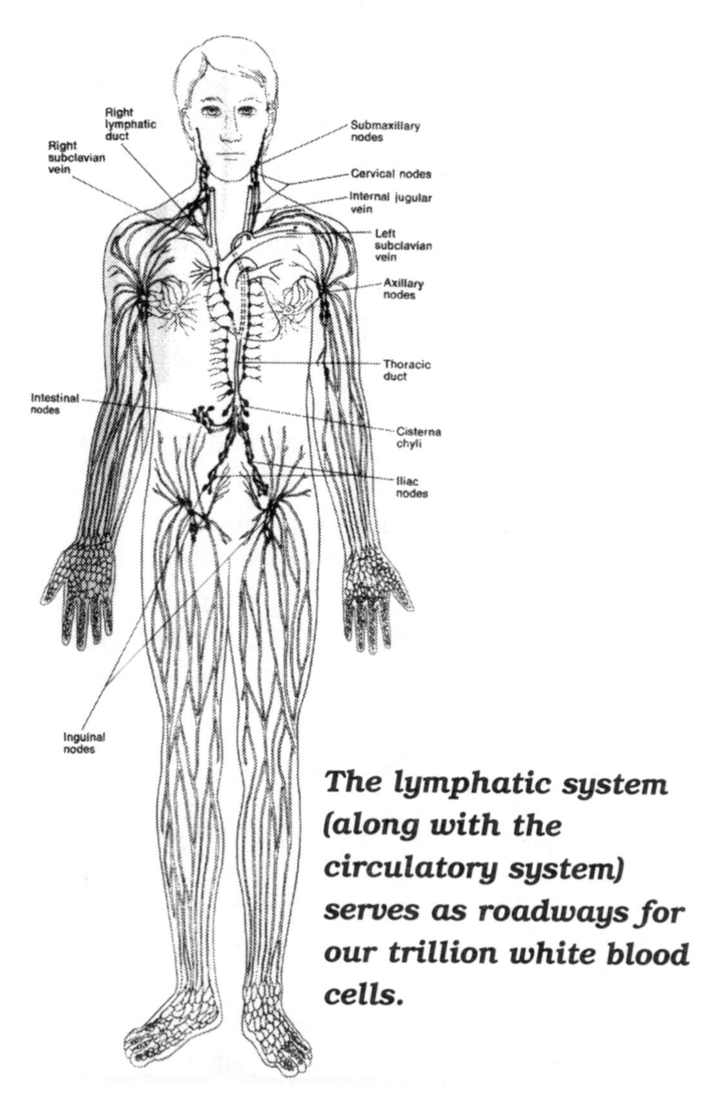

The lymphatic system (along with the circulatory system) serves as roadways for our trillion white blood cells.

There are probably a trillion white blood cells (also called lymphocytes) circulating in the body at all times, or about 3,000 of them in every drop of blood. Over 1,000,000 are created and destroyed every minute. The lymphatic and circulatory systems serve as "roadways" for the elements of the immune system to travel through the body.

The primary objective of these cells is to recognize and attack all substances seen as foreign and to preserve those seen as self. Everything that they don't feel belongs in the body is attacked.

Any substance capable of triggering an immune response is called an antigen. An antigen can be a virus, a bacterium, a fungus, a parasite or even a portion or product of one of these organisms. Tissues or cells from another individual, except an identical twin whose cells carry identical self-markers, also act as antigens; because the immune system recognizes transplanted tissues as foreign, it rejects them. The body will even reject nourishing proteins unless they are first broken down by the digestive system into their primary, non-antigenic building blocks.

The skin is often our first line of defense as it serves as a physical barrier against bacterial, viral or chemical invasion. Body openings such as the oral and nasal cavities, gastrointestinal (GI) tract, genitourinary tract and respiratory tract are guarded against attack by the mucosa rich in lactoferrin, powerful proteolytic enzymes and secretory antibodies that can immobilize and/or destroy invading antigens. Lactoferrin is the first line of defense for any opening in the body. Often there are inadequate amounts of lactoferrin to adequately protect these areas.

When visiting a doctor, the first part of the examination is to observe the oral cavity. "Say ahh."

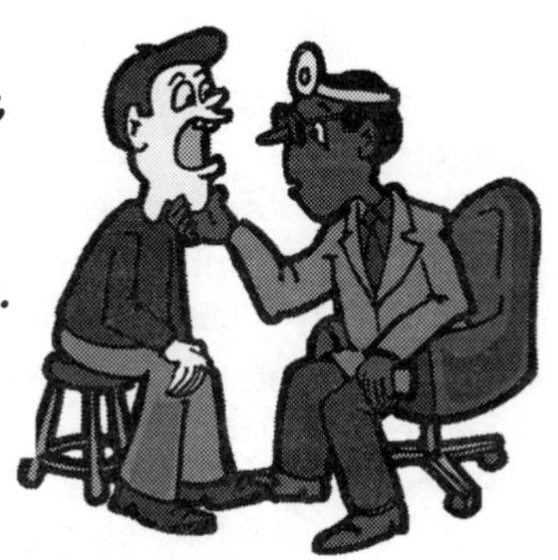

Importance of the Oral Cavity

The importance of the oral cavity as part of the immune system cannot be over stressed. Most infectious micoorganisms enter the body through the oral cavity – inhale them through our nose, mouth or are ingested.

A sore throat is often the first sign of an oncoming cold. As we inhale a cold virus, it may attempt to latch onto it's new host by setting up housekeeping by replicating right there in the back of our throat. As our white blood cells identify it as foreign and alert other white blood cells to rush in to destroy the newly forming colony. We can usually feel the effects of this "battle" as the sensitive tissues in the back of the throat become irritated and inflamed. If the virus is able to replicate enough it will move on - most likely into the sinus and nasal passages. If our immune system is still unsuccessful to combat it, the infection will possibly infiltrate the respiratory system, the lungs.

To prevent the virus (or any other pathogen) from going any further than it's initial place of entrance, the oral cavity is specially designed with mucus membranes and salivary glands. The salivary glands secrete several powerful important immune components including essential mucus, lactoferrin and enzymes like amylase and lysozyme. Immune cells in the mucus tissues also release secretory IgA.

Individuals who have diminished salivary secretion (called dry mouth or xerostomia) have diminished protection against pathogens entering the mouth. Colostrum and lactoferrin lozenge or liquid supplementation can help to counteract this problem.

The oral cavity is loaded with receptor sites which when activated, alert the entire body through a complex chain reaction of immune system events.

To maintain good health, it is critical that we are able to combat disease-causing organisms in the oral cavity before they travel further.

The Mucosal Layer Protects the GI Tract

The GI tract is normally well protected from attack by antigens in ingested food. Often the GI tract's layer of protection will break down leaving us open to pathogens. The mucosal epithelial layer is the interface between the external and internal environments in the gastrointestinal tract. This is the site for the digestion and absorption of most essential nutrients. The mucosal layer also functions as a barrier that prohibits these internal bacteria from entering the rest of the body. The tissue of the intestines is defended by various resistance factors including lactoferrin, that regulates the growth of bacteria in the intestine and assists the body in maintaining its mucosal layer of protection.

A system of lymph nodes, called Peyer's patches, contains cells that secrete various types of white blood cells and IgA, the class of antibodies which protects us from parasitic and microbial invasion.

When bacteria successfully enter the body, they use nutrients supplied by the host to rapidly reproduce and thrive. Just as rapidly, circulating components of the immune system identify the invaders and an immediate attack is initiated against them.

The immune system alerts the body when it identifies a foreign invader by sending a signal and is also responsible for cleaning up after the invader has been conquered. Antibodies form and specialized white blood cells begin to remove the unwelcome substance.

Neutrophils, for example, rush to the site of the invasion and open up to release lactoferrin as the first line of defense. The immune system removes denatured proteins and used-up tissues from the body. If aged red blood cells were not removed each day, one could not survive for more than a few weeks because the blood stream would choke itself with all these useless particles. If just a teaspoon of the iron contained in red blood cells were available to bacteria, they would multiply and fill a large swimming pool in just 24 hours.

Specialized White Blood Cells

These hard-working defenders, which includes the B-Cells, T-Cells, killer T-Cells, suppressor T-Cells and macrophages, have a common objective to destroy all substances, living or inert, that are not naturally part of the human body. These foreign substances can be derived from various sources: microscopic pollens; food allergens such as milk or wheat; other allergens such as dust or animal dander; internally produced substances, even cancerous cells; denatured proteins; and bacteria, viruses and fungi, such as Candida Albicans. If the immune system is weak, the common cold virus or ordinary pollen can become as dangerous as the sting of a scorpion.

B-Cells: These cells search out, identify and bind with specific intruders. B-cells reside in the spleen and lymph nodes and are responsible for production and secretion of antibodies.

T-Cells: These cells form killer T-cells, suppressor T-cells and helper T-cells. Such cells are specialized in killing cells of the body that have been invaded by foreign organisms, as well as cells that have become cancerous. They migrate to the invading microorganisms and destroy the them.

Killer T-Cells: These cells migrate to where antigens are present, attach and destroy the antigens.

Helper T-Cells: These cells identify enemies and rush to the spleen and lymph nodes where they stimulate the production of other cells to fight the infection. They "activate" the killer T-cells.

Suppressor T-Cells: These cells slow down or stop the activities of B-cells and other T-cells, playing a vital role in calling off an attack after an infection has been encountered.

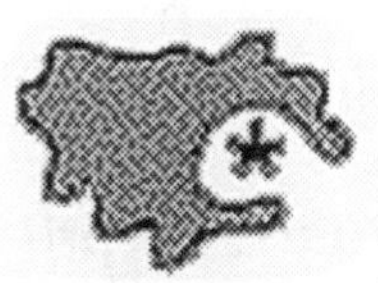

Macrophages: These "scavenger cells" engulf bacteria or cellular debris throughout the body by the process of phagocytosis. They also alert T-cells to the invaders' identities so they can initiate a response, and therefore play a crucial role in initiating the immune response. Macrophages are vital to the regulation of immune responses and inflammation; they churn out an amazing array of powerful chemical substances including enzymes, complement proteins, and regulatory factors such as interleukin-1. At the same time, they carry receptors for lymphokines that allow them to be "activated" into single-minded pursuit of microbes and tumor cells.

Macrophages are strategically located throughout body tissues in a variety of locations. Specialized macrophages include alveolar macrophages in the lungs, mesangial phagocytes in the kidneys, microglial cells in the brain and Kupffer cells in the liver.

As phagocytes, which literally means "cell eater," macrophages rid the body of worn-out cells and other debris. They are large white cells that can engulf and digest microorganisms and other antigenic particles. Some phagocytes also have the ability to present antigens to lymphocytes.

Monocytes: Also considered phagocytes, neutrophils circulate in the blood, then migrate into tissues where they develop into macrophages ("big eaters").

Neutrophils: Neutrophils are not only phagocytes but also granulocytes: they contain granules filled with potent chemicals. These chemicals, in addition to destroying microorganisms, play a key role in acute inflammatory reactions.

Antibodies

Antibodies, also called immunoglobulins, are protein molecules commonly produced in response to the presence of an antigen. Antibodies target a specific invader. They go to the infection site where they either neutralize the enemy (antigen) or tag it for attack by other cells or chemicals.

Antibodies are effective killers within the immune system. Once established, they can clone themselves whenever they are needed to fight off that particular antigen or illness again.

There are five classes of antibodies

IgG: Enhances phagocytosis to neutralize toxins (80 to 85% of total antibody serum).

IgM: Enhances phagocytosis, especially against microorganisms (5 to 10%).

IgA: Protects mucosal surfaces (about 15%).

IgD: Stimulates B-cells to produce antibodies (.2%).

IgE: Associated with allergic reactions (.002%).

We are all provided a genetically active immune system and an acquired immune response. This means part of our immunity is inherited and the rest if obtained through accumulated responses to foreign body exposures.

Immune Protection Against Bacterial and Viral Infection

Most infectious microorganisms enter the body through the mouth and are swallowed. We are confronted constantly with a multitude of various microorganisms every single day. Bacteria are readily found in meat and other animal products, including eggs. Bacteria and microorganisms thrive on improperly cleaned eating utensils and in tap water. Viruses thrive on cold hard surfaces such as bathroom sinks and door handles. We are confronted with microorganisms every time we open a door or use another person's phone, not to mention shaking someone's hand. An unbelievable number of organisms thrive under the fingernails. You may have heard about how unhealthy the air is in airplanes and in office buildings.

Our ability to defend ourselves against these invaders that surround us depends on the health of our immune system. This, of course, is dynamic and depends largely on diet, but also adequate rest, exercise, personal hygiene, smoking, alcohol and drug use and stress.

Normally our immune system is able to properly fight these off and we do not even know it is happening. Some people are not so lucky. Some people catch every cold and bacterial infection that comes their way. Bacterial infections are often treated with antibiotics, which leads to new complications. Antibiotics are also responsible for creating new and unusual challenges for the immune systems of all of us.

Role of Antibiotics

Antibiotics are the perfect example of a good and necessary tool of modern medicine that has been misused to the point where serious problems have evolved. Antibiotics are designed to kill bacteria. The healthy body is teeming with bacteria ("good" and "bad") living together throughout the body.

Problem #1: Some physicians have fallen into the unforgivable habit of prescribing antibiotics for every runny nose, sore throat, earache, or cough that enters the office. Between 80–90% of these ailments are caused by viral infections and an antibiotic is not going to do any good.

Mosty of are not happy unless the doctor gives us a prescription or a shot. Are we satisfied paying a $130.00 office call if all the doctor says is to go home, rest and drink lots of fluids?

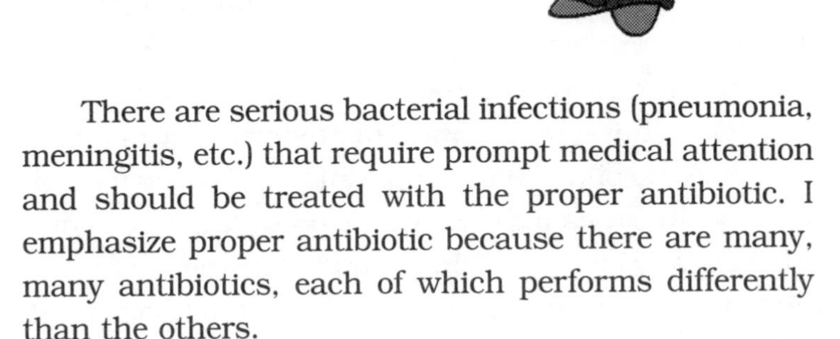

There are serious bacterial infections (pneumonia, meningitis, etc.) that require prompt medical attention and should be treated with the proper antibiotic. I emphasize proper antibiotic because there are many, many antibiotics, each of which performs differently than the others.

The key is to deal with the problem without wrecking total havoc on the rest of the body. Penicillin and erthromycin are thought to attack mainly the "strep" and pneumonia bacteria in the nose, throat and lungs (although they can disrupt vaginal and digestive bacteria as well). Broad spectrum antibiotics such as Keflex®, Ceclor®, ampicillin, amoxicillin, Sepra® and Bactrim®, are not specific and kill all bacteria, disrupting the normal harmonious relationship in the body.

When this relationship is disrupted, yeasts (Candida albicans), normally held in check by bacteria, multiply to undesirable levels. Anyone who has ever suffered with a yeast infection is cautious about altering the balance of their bacterial flora, not wanting to experience it ever again.

Problem #2: In 1998, half of the 53 billion pounds of antibiotics consumed in the United States were fed to farm animals. Antibiotics are often given to the livestock as a preventative. The result is that the natural bacteria living in the animal's intestinal tract (which were harmless) mutate and develop resistance to the antibiotic. These drug-resistant forms of bacteria are currently the cause of up to one-fourth of all bacterial illnesses in the United States. (NEJM, 1984)

The results of eating meat contaminated with antibiotic-resistant bacteria are much more serious and more difficult to treat medically than are the results of eating meat contaminated with normal bacteria. For some, the symptoms include stomach cramps, diarrhea and other food poisoning-like symptoms. Many people simply think they have the 24-hour flu, not even realizing they have food poisoning. (As much as 50% of what we call stomach flu is actually from antibiotic-induced bacterial contaminated meat.) For individuals who might be slightly immuno-compromised, the contamination can be deadly. Children, the elderly and immuno-compromised individuals are especially at risk.

We experienced this in the 1992 "fast-food hamburger tragedy." The culprit, identified as E. coli 0157 is not an ordinary bacteria. It was a prophylactic antibiotic-created "monster-bacteria."

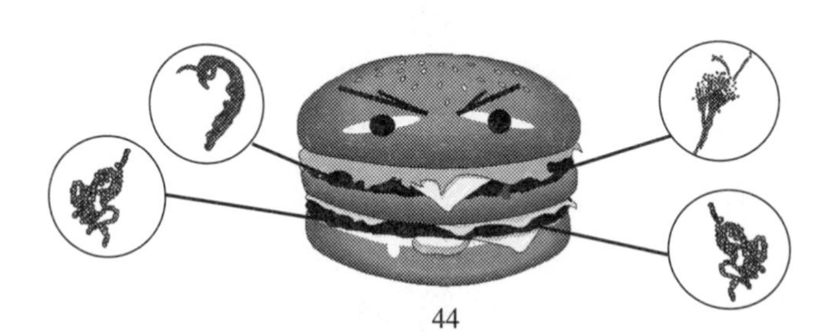

COLOSTRUM

Colostrum is the pre-milk fluid produced by female mammals in the mammary glands just before they give birth. While it is technically not milk at all, colostrum is often called "first milk" as it is obtained in the first milking after birth. Birth is the triggering event that ceases colostrum production in the mother and signals the body for the milk to come in or for the mammal "to freshen".

Colostrum is the fluid held in the mammary tissue until either the:

1) Newborn nurses
2) Mother reabsorbs the nutrients or
3) The colostrum is harvested

After the first milking, the fluid begins to change into milk, containing less colostrum and more milk as time passes. This transitional period lasts 2-3 days. This fluid is referred to as transitional milk.

In all other mammals other than humans, colostrum is crucial to the survival of the newborn. This is because of the high concentration of immuno factors that are transferred through the colostrum. In humans only, some immunofactors are transferred through the placenta. The colostrum is still very important, but if the newborn baby does not receive the colostrum, death is not eminent, as it is in all other mammals. (Hadorn)

TIMING is also very important. If the calf, foal, puppy, etc. experiences difficulties at birth and is unable to nurse for 12 to 18 hours, it will probably die. This is due to the re-absorption of immuno-factors by the mother. It is actually more humane and beneficial for the newborn for the colostrum to be harvested as soon as practical after birth and then bottle-fed to the newborn for the first day of life. (It is more sanitary for livestock to be bottle-fed at this sensitive stage.) This allows the newborn to receive excellent quality colostrum during the critical first 24 hours of life. Unless the colostrum is harvested immediately after birth, the quality is greatly compromised.

When selecting a colostrum supplement, it is important to keep the time of collection in mind. Also note that in virtually every scientific study performed on colostrum, the researchers diligently pursue the

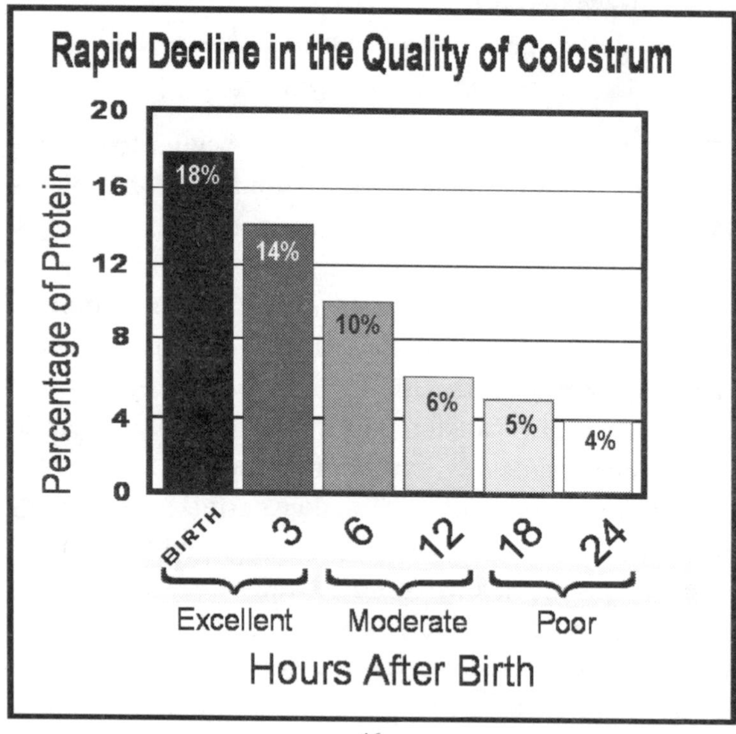

highest quality they can obtain at the time of the study. Research results indicate that both the quality of the colostrum and method of delivery (into the oral cavity) are very important.

Keep in mind that all of the nutritional benefits (vitamins, minerals, essential fatty acids, etc.) of breast milk and colostrum are not really applicable to supplemental forms. Breast milk is the infants only food and they may consume several pints a day. The small amount of colostrum in a supplement does not supply adequate amounts of these nutrients for an adult. The focus of colostrum as a supplement is the immunofactors, which are not required in huge amounts to stimulate and support the immune system.

Breast Milk: A Perfect Food

In humans as well as other mammals, a newborn's very first meal of colostrum is of great significance to its health and well being for the rest of its life. The immune system of the newborn is not fully developed, making it highly susceptible to numerous pathogens, antigens and allergens. Colostrum provided in breast milk contains all the needed immune factors that are essential to activate, regulate and balance the immune system. This is of great significance as the newborn's own system develops.

Mother's milk provides the perfectly assigned, individualized nutritional food to promote passive immunity and proper growth and development. As mammals grow, essential glycoproteins in breast milk keep the immune system functional.

Nutritional Support + Immunity

Mother's milk provides both immunity (passive and active) and nutritional benefits. The lipids, carbohydrates, amino acids and other nutrients provide the baby with ideal nutrition and, therefore, enhance the overall health of the baby. Colostrum provides rich immune factors to sensitive newborns who cannot yet fend for themselves. Peyer's patches, found throughout the intestinal tract, and groups of immunoactive cells in the bronchial mucosa that destroy allergens, antigens and pathogens, are not yet operative in the newborn.

Colostrum contains antibodies against E. coli, Salmonella, Shigella. V. cholera, Bacteriodes fragilis, Streptococcus pneumonia, Bordtella pertussis, Clostridium diphtheria, Streptococcus Mutans, Clostridium tetani and Candida albicans. (Ogra)

Beast-feeding was also found to be effective against the hepatitis C virus (HCV). Research shows that both anti-HCV antibody and HCV-ribonucleic acid are present in colostrum. (Lin)

Other infections prevented by breast feeding:

Respiratory infections
Respiratory syncytial virus
Haemophilus influenza
Enterovirus
Enteric infections
Polio virus
Rotavirus
Cryptosporidium parvum (Goldblum)

Babies deprived of breast milk are simply not as healthy as those who are breast-fed. Nonbreast-fed babies develop eczema, food and upper respiratory allergies and gastrointestinal problems at a much higher rate than breast-fed babies do. (Juto)

Acquired maternal antibodies are also transferred through breast feeding and will protect the baby. For example, if the mother has contracted a disease such as measles, pertussis, or mumps, sometime prior to pregnancy, she has developed antibodies against them making her immune to reinfection. These antibodies are passed on in her breast milk to protect the baby from contracting these conditions while breast feeding. This is a most critical time of growth and development. Breast-fed babies who do contract these conditions later will experience a milder condition with far fewer complications compared to nonbreast-fed babies.

Mother's milk supplies:

Immunoglobulins: Breast milk contains all five types of antibodies (IgG, IgM, IgD, IgE, and IgA), which fight off bacteria, viruses, allergens and yeast. Each has a specific function in the immune system. Colostrum contains the highest concentration of these immunoglobulins.

These antibodies in colostrum also provide specific defense to fight microorganisms that cause polio, pneumonia, dysentery, candidiasis and many others.

Secretory IgA makes up 90% of the immunoglobulins in human milk. This specifically protects the baby against enteric pathogens such as E. coli. Lactoferrin has been shown to increase secretory IgA and to protect the GI tract from invasion from such pathogens. (Kruzel)

Leukocytes: Living white blood cells consisting mostly of macrophages and neutrophils. T-cells are also present.

Accessory Factors: Including peroxidase enzymes which destroy disease-carrying microorganisms by oxidation, and also lactoferrin and polysaccharldes which neutralize some strains of bacteria. Many disease-carrying microorganisms do not survive well in an oxygenated environment. Also, cancer cells thrive in an anaerobic (non-oxygen) environment.

PRP (Proline-Rich-Polypeptides): A special regulatory polypeptide that calms the immune system when overactive, and stimulates it when underactive.

Interferon: Inhibits viral activity.

Lactobacillus Bifidus: Beneficial bacteria naturally occurring in the lower intestines that prevents the overgrowth of dangerous bacteria. It also helps keep the Candida albicans fungus under control.

Lactoferrin: An extremely important iron-binding protein in milk. Lactoferrin interferes in the growth of potentially harmful bacteria in the intestine. Many functions have been attributed to lactoferrin, including antimicrobial and antiviral activities, immunomodulation and cell growth regulation. Lactoferrin enhances phagocytosis, cell adherence and controls the release of proinflammatory cytokines such as IL-1, IL-6 and TNF-alpha. Lactoferrin also diminishes the damaging effects of free radicals.

Coenzyme: A protein which is thought not to be digested, but to persist in the gastrointestinal tract where it breaks down the cell walls of certain unwanted bacteria, preventing their proliferation.

Lactalbumins: Proteins which are easier for the infant to digest than the casein proteins of non-heat-treated cows milk.

Lactose: Main carbohydrate in human (and animal) milk. It promotes the absorption of calcium and some other minerals. As colostrum diminishes and is replaced by milk, the levels of lactose increase.

Oligosaccharides: Carbohydrate component which allows proliferation of healthy intestinal bacteria and interferes with the adherence of undesirable microorganisms.

Transforming Growth Factor (TGF): Responsible for normal cell growth and repair. Important for rapid growth and development of newborn.

Nucleotides: Raw materials needed to build and repair the vital DNA and RNA of the cell.

Vitamins: Breast milk is a rich source of vitamins A, E and B-12, and also contains adequate amounts of vitamin D and pro-vitamin A, beta carotene. In addition to the antioxidant effects, vitamin E stimulates the development of immunity in the newborn.

Minerals: These are suited to the infant's needs to facilitate absorption. The iron in breast milk is highly absorbable by the infant. (Christan, Wootan)

Anti-inflammatory agents: Breast milk provides a number of components that fight off inflammation: Antimicrobial factors (Secretory IgA. lactoferrin, lysozyme), antioxidants (vitamins A and E, and beta carotene), enzymes that break down inflammatory mediators, anti-enzymes, cytoprotective agents and modulators of leukocyte activation. (Goldblum)

Taurine for Brain Development: Among other amino acids, breast milk contains high amounts of taurine, which is crucial for the regulation of cell growth. Brain development seems to be the most important. In humans 95% of all brain development in humans takes place before age five. Interestingly, the average age for infant-led weaning in countries where it is allowed to naturally occur is five years. Taurine deficiency has resulted in growth retardation in monkeys. Retinal development in the eye is also highly significant. (Wootan)

Lipids: Fatty acids supply half of the kilocalories in breast milk. Their triglyceride structure makes them highly absorbable. Cholesterol makes up a large portion of the fats in breast milk and colostrum, providing six times more cholesterol than formula. This cholesterol is needed for structural development.

Essential Fatty Acids (EFAs): Linoleic (LA), Linolenic (LNA) and Docosahexaenoic (DHA) Acids are crucial for cognitive and visual development. In the early 1990's, many formula developers began supplementing formulas with LA and LNA. Unfortunately, it was later revealed that infants were unable to effectively convert LNA into DHA, and thus were still deficient compared to breast-fed babies. Preformed DHA must be provided since the body during these periods is unable to make it. (Cockburn, Carlson, Neuringer)

Higher IQ/Fewer Neurological Problems

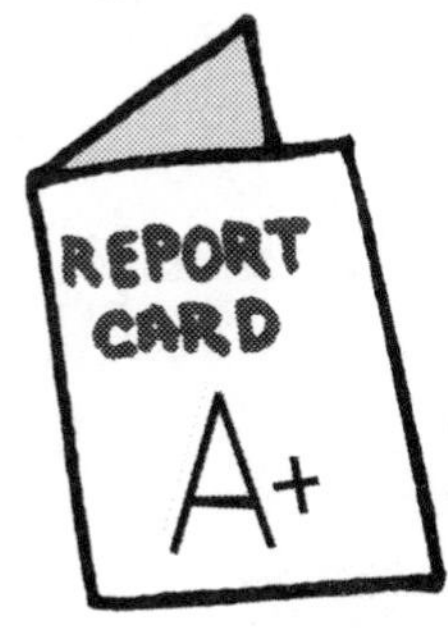

Numerous studies have reported that children who had consumed mother's milk in the early weeks of life had a significantly higher IQ at seven and one-half and eight years of age than those who received none. The researchers found that the longer the child consumed breast milk, the higher the child's IQ.

Breast-fed infants are also known to be more active and to pass their motor milestones earlier than formula-fed babies without DHA. (Taylor, Fergusson)

Also interesting is that children who never received breast milk were perceived as having worse behavior (at five years old) than breast-fed infants. (Taylor) Another study found that infants who were not breast-fed were twice as likely to have neurological disfunction, which often contributes to behavioral and learning difficulties in school. IQ deficits and neurological disfunction are considered risk factors for criminal behavior. (Crime Times)

Protection from Allergies, Inflammatory and Autoimmune Diseases

Autoantibodies in colostrum serum play a major role in the selection of the pre-immune B-cell repertoire and in the maintenance of the immune homeostasis. Researchers hypothesize that the natural autoantibodies in colostrum and milk may contribute to the selection process of physiological development during the early postnatal period in breast-fed infants. This could explain the lower frequency of allergic, inflammatory, autoimmune diseases and lymphomas which are seen in individuals who were breast-fed as infants. (Vassilev)

Colostrum Benefits Infants with Diarrhea

Studies report colostrum helps manage infants with chronic diarrhea. In eight children with chronic diarrhea, ranging from nine months to three years of age, E. coli was present in all eight cases, Ascaris lambricoidis in four, and Giardia lambia in one. All eight children were given 20 ml. fresh human colostrum daily for seven days. In addition, those who had giardiasis received metronidazole treatment, while cases with ascariasis were given antihelminthic therapy. The results indicated that colostrum provided effective antidiarrheal action in some patents with chronic diarrhea of infective origin. (Saha)

Growth Factors

The effects of human colostrum in promoting baby growth and development are much stronger than they are in human milk or bovine colostrum.

Studies show the activity of human colostrum in stimulating DNA synthesis was 20 times greater than that of bovine serum. The activity of growth factors in human colostrum was higher than that in human milk or bovine colostrum, and only human colostrum contains two different kinds of growth factors: CAGF, an epidermal growth factor, and CBGF, a platelet differentiation growth factor. (Ye)

Promotes Development of Infant GI Tract

Following birth, the infant gastrointestinal tract (esophagus, stomach and small intestine) undergoes profound growth, changes and functional maturation. Epithelial cells in the small intestines lose the ability to absorb macromolecules, and the epithelial cells of the large intestine lose the ability to synthesize digestive enzymes and to absorb amino acids and glucose.

These changes are apparently related to the onset of colostrum ingestion, because starved or water-fed newborns showed little changes in the GI tract. This is due to the hormones and growth-promoting peptides, such as insulin, cortisol, epidermal growth factor (EGF) and insulin-like growth factor I (IGF-I) found at high concentrations in the maternal colostrum.

Human colostrum, contains high concentrations of motilin and gastrin (hormones that stimulate the flow of gastric juices and cause bile and pancreatic enzyme release). Motilin and gastrin concentrations in human colostrum are the highest compared to human mature milk, cow colostrum and cow mature milk. The difference in motilin concentration was very significant between human milk and cow milk. (Lu)

These component in colostrum can also be used therapeutically for premature infants or newborns with immature or diseased GI tracts. (Xu)

Every mother wants the best for her child. When breast feeding is not an option, colostrum and lactoferrin are still available.

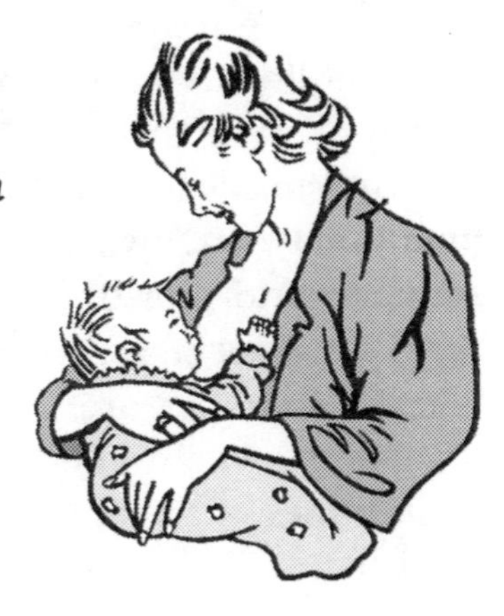

Breast Milk Linked to Low Cholesterol

Breast-fed babies may be less likely to have elevated cholesterol levels as adults. A researcher at Baylor College of Medicine in Houston says a study of four-month-olds found differences in the way formula-fed infants produce cholesterol, which is crucial for the brain's development.

Breast milk has six times more cholesterol than formula, and formula-fed babies respond by producing their own, says Dr. William Wong, Associate Professor of Pediatrics at Baylor. Despite the increased production, formula-fed babies still have 40% less cholesterol in their blood. Wong suggests that the formula-fed infants are receiving inadequate cholesterol causing them to produce it. This increased cholesterol production during infancy may have an "imprinting effect" that persists later in life, meaning that formula-fed babies may suffer from higher cholesterol levels as adults. (Butte, Wong)

So Perfect Only Nature Could Think of It

Colostrum is highly beneficial in the unique manner in which it provides the body with its numerous immune factors in the mouth, stomach and intestinal tract. The entire digestive tract starting with the oral cavity is lined with mucous membranes. Most infectious microorganisms enter the body through the mouth (especially true for infants) or respiratory tract (many are swallowed). The mucosal surfaces of the stomach and intestinal tracts are where most infectious diseases become localized. To remain healthy, it is critical that we are able to combat disease-causing organisms where they attack us, on the mucous membranes of the oral cavity, stomach and intestinal tract.

Colostrum is specially designed to protect us because most of the antibodies' other immune factors provided in colostrum are not digested and absorbed, but remain in the intestinal tract where they are able to fight off invaders.

Final Comments on Immunity in Children

U.S. children are often said to have poor health status compared to children in the rest of the world. One of the main reasons is the lack of breast-feeding.

While a lack of immunizations has been blamed, it is hardly relevant. Pediatric medical authorities such as Dr. George Wootan states, "O*ne needs to look at the frequency of these diseases prior to the introduction of the immunizations. When one looks at the statistics today, one sees the previous high incidence of deaths from these diseases while today we have a low incidence of those deaths. People assume that the reason is because of the vaccines now available.*"

"*The decline of approximately 90% of the diseases (whooping cough. measles, tetanus, diphtheria, small pox, polio, etc.) took place before the advent of significant medical advances and before the vaccines came to exist. To give the vaccines the whole credit (while they do deserve some) for the disease decline is not correct.*"

"*The economic well-being of the pharmaceutical companies who manufacture the vaccines is very much responsible for our current beliefs about health issues, and much of what they want us to believe is incorrect and/or misleading.*"

Recommended reading: *Take Charge of Your Child's Health*, George Wootan, M.D., Crown Publishers, Inc., New York 1992.

COLOSTRUM AS A SUPPLEMENT FOR INFANTS AND CHILDREN

I Could Not Breast-Feed – What Now?

Ideally, women should breast-feed as long as possible. But life is not always "ideal." Some women are unable to breast-feed their newborn or cannot breast feed for the entire first year due to mastitis or other reasons. The benefits of colostrum can still be obtained through colostrum supplementation. By supplementing your bottle-fed child with an excellent quality, pure, unadulterated, liquid bovine colostrum, it is still possible to obtain many of the immuno and growth factors so important for proper development.

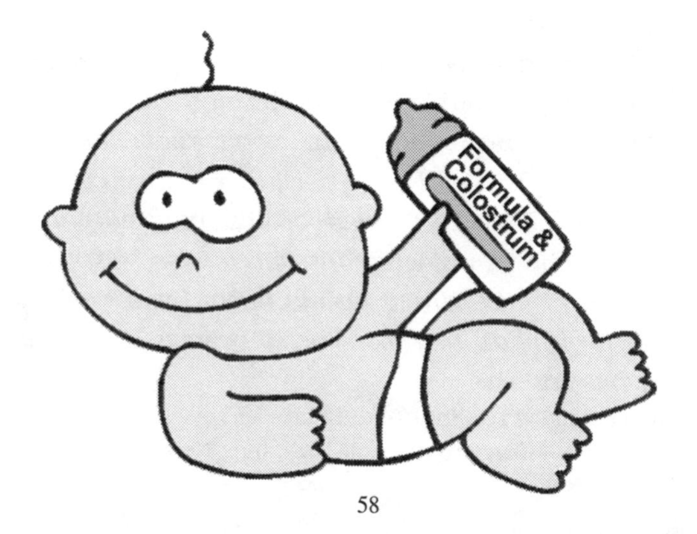

If the following regime is adhered to each time your infant drinks, you will help to ensure proper immunity, brain and gastrointestinal development for your infant. This is an excellent way to supplement the diet for infants that are unable to breast-feed.

Please note that the following is only applicable for excellent quality bovine colostrum liquid. Suggested use for any other quality colostrum cannot be predicted nor can the results.

Colostrum Liquid Supplementation for Infants

Birth to 6 Months: Add 1 drop/day in formula, water or juice. If the infant is in any type of distress, add 1 drop/feeding until distress is gone and then continue 1 drop/day.

6 Months to 1 Year: Add 2 drops/day in formula, water or juice. If the infant is in any type of distress, add 2 drops/feeding until distress is gone and then continue 2 drops/day.

Over 1 Year: Add 3 drops/day for each year of age. If in distress, use 3 drops/feeding for each year of age.

After age two, or when the child is old enough, you can start them on a regime of lozenges to continue the process. Excellent quality lozenges are available through most fine health food stores. If you can find a product that combines both colostrum and lactoferrin in an oral delivery it will save time and effort while providing the best for your child.

Colostrum and Milk: A Comparison

Colostrum and milk are very different and for all practical purposes, there is no reason to compare them, but here are the major differences:

Over 37 different beneficial immune factors have been identified in colostrum. There are increasing numbers of studies that show it is helpful in combating viral infections in general. A major Australian study reported in *The Lancet* showed that bovine colostrum protected children against retrovirus, the major cause of infectious diarrhea in children. None of the 55 children given colostrum contracted diarrhea.

Colostrum provides high levels of immunoglobulins, with a wide range of specific antibodies against bacteria, viruses and the yeast normally present in the gastrointestinal tract. This prevents the colonization of pathogens and toxin generation. This, in turn, is protective to the body.

Colostrum also contains immune regulatory factors, which are called biogenic simulators. These are known to promote cell growth, tissue repair, healing and normalization.

Fortunately, the numerous immune factors found in colostrum are transferrable from one species to another. This means that humans can benefit from the immune-rich colostrum from cows.

Colostrum from cows is much richer in immune factors than that of humans. (Sandholm) Human colostrum contains only 2% IgG (the body's most important immunoglobulin) while bovine colostrum contains 86% IgG. (Bunce)

As a liquid, cow's milk contains approximately 4% protein (80% casein and only 10% immunoglobulins). At birth, colostrum contains almost 20% protein, yet quickly degrades to just 4% in 24 hours. *(See the chart on page 46.)* Approximately 55% of this is immunoglobulins.

When colostrum is properly harvested and dried, it should contain at least 50% protein. Immunoglobulins will then be at least 40% of the protein content. True colostrum will be obtained before being diluted with milk. Typically this will require milking within the first 6 hours after birth.

Bovine-derived colostrum has several differences and advantages over typical milk:

1. It is higher in protein and antibodies.

2. It is higher in vitamins and minerals.

3. It is lower in fat and sugar.

4. It contains significant amounts of immune factors: Immunoglobulins, accessory factors, polypeptides, transforming growth factor, nucleotides, antibody-stimulating factors, hormones, vitamins, minerals, nucleotides, enzymes and various non-immunoglobulin components that destroy disease-causing microorganisms.

Cow's Milk Is for Cows, Not For Babies

The late Benjamin Spock, M.D., author of *Dr. Spock's Baby and Child Care*, was renowned as one of the world's foremost expert pediatricians for close to 50 years. Together with the Physicians Committee for Responsible Medicine (PCRM), Dr. Spock warned that milk can cause health problems. Frank Oski, M.D., the Director of Pediatrics at Johns Hopkins University and author of the revolutionary book, *Don't Drink Your Milk,* and Neal Barnard, M.D., President of PCRM, are just a few others who contend that cow's milk is certainly not nature's perfect food, at least for humans.

The PCRM recommends feeding breast milk at least until infants are age one. After that, they stated that there is no nutritional need for cow's milk in the diets of human children or adults.

"Cow's milk in the past has always been oversold as the perfect food," commented Dr. Spock, *"but we are now seeing that it isn't the perfect food at all and the government really shouldn't be behind any efforts to promote it as such. At the press conference, it was*

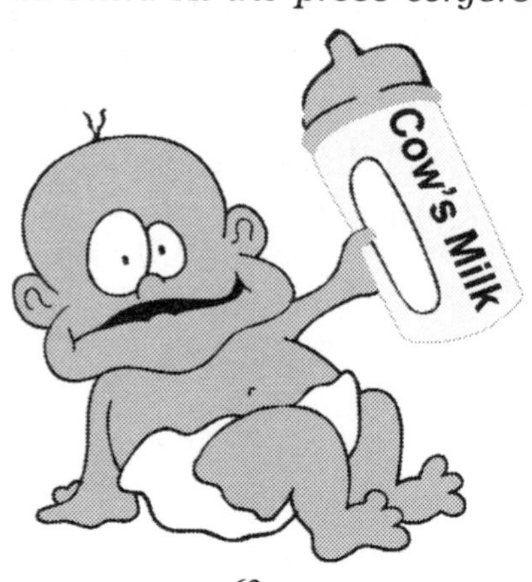

not my intention to announce that cow's milk is bad for all children and adults, although this may have been the consensus of the other members of the group. As a parent educator for many, many years. it has been my job to interpret the latest ever-changing stages of available knowledge and I now want to express my concern on behalf of the recent details available concerning cow's milk for some people."

"We really want to stress the fact that mothers who give their children milk and dairy products should not feel guilty, but milk is not a required part of the diet and children can be raised healthy without it. And, in fact, evidence is showing that we all may be healthier without it," said Spock.

What's Wrong with Milk and Dairy Products?

According to the PCRM, there are a whole host of specific problems identified with dairy products today for both adults and children.

1. Cow's milk can cause iron-deficiency anemia.

The first concern addressed at the PCRM was anemia, which is especially prevalent in children. For this reason, the American Academy of Pediatrics recommended in 1992 that whole milk not be given to infants less than one year of age. They stated that milk is so low in iron that an infant would have to drink more than 31 quarts of milk per day in order to get the D.V. of 15 mg. iron. In addition, milk can cause blood loss from the intestinal tract, depleting the body's iron. The reason for this tendency is unclear.

Despite the fact that breast milk actually contains less iron than cow's milk, breast milk iron is 100% absorbable compared to 30% absorbable in cow's milk.

2. Cow's milk may trigger diabetes.

The PCRM also brought up the fact that milk has been implicated as a trigger for insulin-dependent diabetes, which affects approximately one million Americans. Diabetes is the cause of half of all leg and foot amputations and causes blindness in 12,000 people annually.

A study published in *The New England Journal of Medicine* reported that a protein in cow's milk causes elevation of antibodies that destroy insulin secreting beta cells in the pancreas in genetically susceptible people, increasing the risk for diabetics.

The study reported that of 142 insulin-dependent children and 79 healthy children, all diabetic children had elevation of specific antibodies to the albumin-containing amino acids in cow's milk. None of the non-diabetic children had elevation of these antibodies.

This is certainly not the first study to demonstrate this link. According to Dr. Barnard, who also wrote *The Power of Your Plate* and *Food For Life*, epidemiological studies show that in countries such as the United States and Finland, where milk consumption beyond infancy is common, there is a 36 times higher incidence of juvenile-onset insulin-dependent diabetes, compared to countries such as Japan, where milk is not normally consumed. Also interesting to note is that the incidence of genetic predisposition in these different countries is about the same, said Dr. Barnard.

3. Cow's milk causes allergies, digestive problems.

Many, many people lack the digestive enzyme lactase necessary to digest dairy products, which contain lactose, milk sugar. This enzyme is produced by the cells that line the small intestine in individuals who seem able to tolerate milk.

According to the National Institute of Diabetes and Digestive and Kidney Diseases, in 1991, 50 million people were lactose intolerant. As many as 75% of all African-American, Jewish, Native American, and Mexican-American adults are lactose intolerant. An estimated 90% of Asian-American adults are lactose intolerant. These individuals suffer from nausea, bloating, painful gas, abdominal cramps and diarrhea.

Many people are allergic to milk protein. Milk protein allergies are among the most common type of food allergy. Allergic reactions to dairy products are extremely varied. A few people experience classical reactions such as hives, rashes, cramps, and anaphylactic-type reactions, but most people experience the non-classical reactions. It is much harder to determine that dairy products are the cause of these reactions unless you do a food elimination test. This type of allergy usually does not show up in the typical skin allergy test (RAST). The reactions include asthma, recurrent bronchial infections, joint pain (arthritis), insomnia, skin problems such as acne and digestive problems such as gas, bloating, stomach pain and nausea. There are medications available for many of these symptoms, and most people choose to simply put up with these reactions all their lives.

Infants are never allergic to mother's milk and breast-fed babies suffer far fewer digestive problems. They are almost never constipated.

COLOSTRUM AS A SUPPLEMENT FOR ADULTS

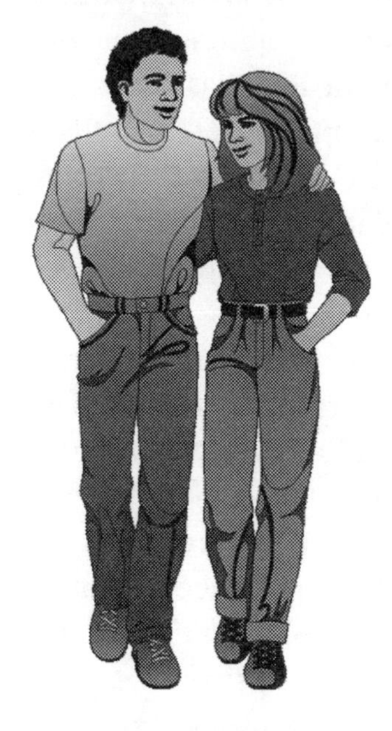

We have explored how a mammal conveys immunity to its newborn, but how did the mother obtain the immunity in the first place? All mammals build immunity during their lifetime based upon the pathogens they come in contact with. If a mammal grows up in a sheltered environment free of toxins and pathogens, its immunity will be much lower than a mammal growing up in close proximity to other mammals and therefore numerous pathogens. You may recall how remote tribes all over the world were all but eliminated when explorers came into their camps and accidentally introduced a common form of influenza. Since the tribes had never encountered the flu, they had no immunity to fight it off.

Back to Basics

For years bovine colostrum has been used as a folk remedy in Scandinavian countries. This changed in the 1950's when all the "highly sophisticated, medically-advanced" miracle drugs came into the picture.

One could experience instant relief from infectious disease. "Just take a pill and you're cured!" (Not really, but that is what we thought.)

People chose to ignore older, traditional methods that clearly worked, but for which there was no clear scientific explanation. The many complicated factors which make up colostrum work together. It does not have just one easy-to-describe mode of action, like penicillin.

New Strains of Bacteria and Viruses

Deadly microbes have learned how to circumvent modern medicine's arsenal of antibiotics and they continue to mutate. Emory University researchers discovered this fact in the diapers of Atlanta day-care kids, in mathematical models and in countless laboratory cultures that have tracked antibiotic resistance traits through thousands of bacterial generations. Amid the rising tide of antibiotic-resistant diseases, from bubonic plague to childhood ear infections, doctors and scientists have taken some comfort in the notion that if antibiotic use could be curbed, the resistant bugs - less fit for antibiotic-free environments than their susceptible cousins - would fade away. "*Technology is losing the arms race with evolution,*" says Professor Bruce Levin, the director of Emory's graduate program in population biology and ecology and evolution. Many scientists believe that the continued widespread use of antibiotics in medicine and agriculture makes increases in resistant microbes inevitable. In the half-century since the development of penicillin, virtually every infectious microbe has developed resistance to one or more of the major classes of antibiotics. (Toner)

Antibiotic-resistant bacteria are not only more difficult to treat than their more drug-susceptible cousins, they can also be more than twice as expensive, according to a limited survey through Duke University Medical Center. (Manning)

Medical research has traditionally been centered on treating illness with medication instead of developing wellness in the entire body. Medications are targeted at a specific ailment without total understanding of the effects they have on our complete system. Often we overcome one illness with medication only to be plagued by another illness. Medication is necessary and desirable at critical times when it is not possible for the body's systems to heal itself. In most non-clinical situations, the best solution is to treat the body and to let the body's systems treat the illness.

Our current medical environment

The prevalence of AIDS, immune disorders such as Lyme disease, Epstein-Barr (chronic infectious mononucleosis, sometimes called Chronic Fatigue Syndrome), fibromyalgia, Candida-Related-Complex, Herpes Simplex and various autoimmune disorders have forced us to learn more about our immune system, our health in general and the effect of negative lifestyles. These immune disorders have caused us to review all the nutritional options. One of these is the use of supplemental colostrum and lactoferrin.

Colostrum was specially designed by nature to:

- ***Protect***
- ***Activate***
- ***Regulate***
- ***Support our immune system***

Protection

Immunoglobulins

Colostrum contains all four of the key immunoglobulins: IgM, IgG, IgA and secretory IgA. These immunoglobulins are equipped with special adaptive sites which are effective at neutralizing a wide range of bacteria, viruses and yeasts. (Brandtzaeg) They include antibodies specific to fight disease-causing microorganisms.

Colostrum provides specific antibody reactivity to bacteria, viruses and yeasts. (Ogra) Most infectious diseases enter the body through the mouth or remain localized in mucosal surfaces, primarily the stomach and intestinal tract. (Weldham) We must be able to combat diseases-causing organisms where they attack us.

Fortunately, colostrum helps us do that. Most of the colostrum antibodies are believed not to be absorbed and digested but to remain in the intestinal tract after being swallowed where they fight off intruders. (Tyrell)

It is commonly assumed that the digestive enzymes in the stomach and intestines would break up or digest the immunoglobulin-protein molecules in colostrum when ingested; Research has shown, however, that colostrum contains a powerful trypsin inhibitor and a number of protease inhibitors that protect the immune factors from breaking up. (Von Fellenberg)

The major benefits of immune factors in colostrum and lactoferrin occur within the mouth, stomach and on the intestinal and bronchial walls, and not as a result of their passage into the tissues. (Tyrell) This means if the majority of immune-enhancing benefits occurs in these locations, colostrum can benefit people of all ages. Added support can make a tremendous difference where the immune system is marginal or below marginal.

Leukocytes (White Blood Cells)

Colostrum contains living white blood cells able to protect us from a variety of pathogens. Neutrophils and macrophages are the most prominent cells in colostrum. Lymphocytes are also present, predominantly T-cells, capable of producing interferon and other protective factors.

Colostrum Offers Safe Viral and Bacterial Protection

Dozens of scientific papers suggest that colostrum can block or reduce the severity of a wide variety of infections including many which have their initiation in the oral/fecal route.

Colostrum is effective against a number of microorganisms including the following bacteria: E. coli (including 0157 strain), Streptococcus pneumococci, Clostridium difficile toxins A and B, Vibrio cholera, Salmonella, Shigella, Bactericide fragilis, Bordtel Ia pertussis, and the following viruses: Rotavirus, Respiratory Syncytial Virus (RSV), Coxsackie, Echo and Alphaviruses, Poliomyelitis, Enteric, Hemagglutinating Encephalitis, Herpes Simplex and yeasts such as Candida albicans.

Escherichia coli

E. coli is a species of bacteria which normally lives in the intestines of humans, and also in the feces of cattle. It is common in water, milk and soil. It is the most frequent cause of urinary tract infections and a cause of serious infection in wounds. E. coli is also responsible for diarrhea, and for the production of toxins that create intestinal irritation because of their ability to adhere to the intestinal wall.

Numerous researchers have demonstrated that colostrum has bacteriostatic and bacteriocidal effects against E. coli. Peroxidase, lactoferrin and IgA, all found in colostrum, are capable of creating powerful effects against E. coli.

Streptococcus pneumonococci

Streptococcus pneumonococci is the cause of 90% of the cases of bacterial pneumonia in the United States. Oligosaccharides found in colostrum have been shown to block attachment of a wide variety of bacteria, especially S. pneumonococci, to mucous membranes, thereby aiding in the prevention of respiratory inflammations. (Hanson)

Clostridium difficile toxins A and B

Clostridium bacteria are spore-forming and need no oxygen to live. The proliferation of this bacteria is believed to be predominantly the result of two toxins. Studies have shown that colostrum is effective in neutralizing these two Clostridium difficile toxins. (Kim)

Salmonella

Salmonella infection is commonly caused by eating contaminated food. Three syndromes caused by Salmonella infection in humans are gastroenteritis (commonly marked by sharp pain in the stomach or intestines, watery diarrhea, nausea and vomiting), and enteric and typhoid fever. (Salmonella can be largely avoided by proper hygiene, proper hand washing, cooking foods adequately and keeping foods in the refrigerator.) Colostrum is effective against Salmonella.

Rotavirus

Rotavirus is probably the most common cause of infant death in developing countries. Studies have shown that colostrum has protective properties against Rotavirus diarrhea outbreak.

After immunizing 8-month pregnant Holstein cows with human rotavirus (Wa strain), the cow colostrum containing neutralizing antibody to human rotavirus was obtained. After randomly grouping 13 infants from a single orphanage, six infants received 20 ml. of Rota hyper-immune colostrum every morning and seven control infants received 20 ml. of market milk.

One month later, rotavirus-associated diarrhea was observed in six of the seven infants given milk and only one out of the six infants given Rota hyper-immune colostrum. Orally administered Rota hyper-immune colostrum significantly protected infants from diarrhea caused by rotavirus. Two out of five Rota hyper-immune colostrum recipients who were free from diarrhea showed rises in antibody titer after the rotavirus infection epidemic.

While the Rota hyper-immune colostrum prevented the outbreak of diarrhea, it did not prevent immunological responses to natural rotavirus infection. In the trial, Rota hyper-immune colostrum had no effect on duration of diarrhea, bowel movements or virus shedding in stool. There were no side effects of Rota hyper-immune colostrum administration (Ebina)

Respiratory Syncytial Virus

This virus is often the cause of bronchitis and pneumonia in humans. In 1982, research at the State University of New York at Buffalo demonstrated that humans and animals exposed to Respiratory Syncytial Virus (RSV) developed protective antibodies against this virus in the IgG and IgA classes. These protective antibodies were found in large quantities in colostrum, particularly those of the IgG class. (Theodore)

Herpes Simplex Virus

Herpes simplex, which is highly contagious, is known to cause cold sores. Since the 1970's we have known that bovine colostrum are able to destroy Herpes simplex virus-infected cells. (Kohl)

I could not locate any specific human studies on the effect of colostrum or lactoferrin supplementation on cold sores, but I suspect that they would decrease one's risk of outbreak as one's immunity would be strengthened.

Candida Albicans

Several studies have revealed that colostrum leukocytes proved to be effective in controlling the yeast infection Candida albicans. (Ho, Goldman)

Researchers in Denmark reported that colostrum tablets proved to be effective treatment for oral Candida among HIV-infected individuals, given ten times a day for ten days. (Christensen)

Bowel irregularity and inconsistency are problems that often accompany intestinal bacterial upset. These problems can be addressed by colostrum powder in capsule form because it tends to promote the growth of bifida bacteria and other healthy flora in the intestinal tract. These beneficial bacteria help maintain a homeostatic environment and help stimulate the musculature of the colon.

A healthy intestinal microbial flora population also promotes an improved and comfortable digestive tract and helps one avoid gas and bloating.

Colostrum promotes a healthy intestinal microflora population, enhances utilization of the nutrients in the foods we eat, and provides protection against enteric pathogens. Therefore, it helps provides a stable, stronger defense against infection by organisms, whether they are bacteria, virus or parasite, which especially seek a weakened host.

Activation

Imagine the activity of the immune system as a complex setup of dominos with numerous extending branches or "arms" which each have their own extending branches and so on. There is one starting point - a point of activation where you simply have to tap the first domino to begin the chain reaction of falling dominos to complete the process.

The oral cavity is this place of activation. The oral cavity is loaded with receptor sites which when activated, alert the entire body through a complex chain reaction of immune system events.

Supplementing colostrum of excellent quality from the first milking in the mucosal membranes of the mouth triggers the chain reaction to occur throughout the body. This excellent quality colostrum can trigger a response that will reach all aspects of the immune

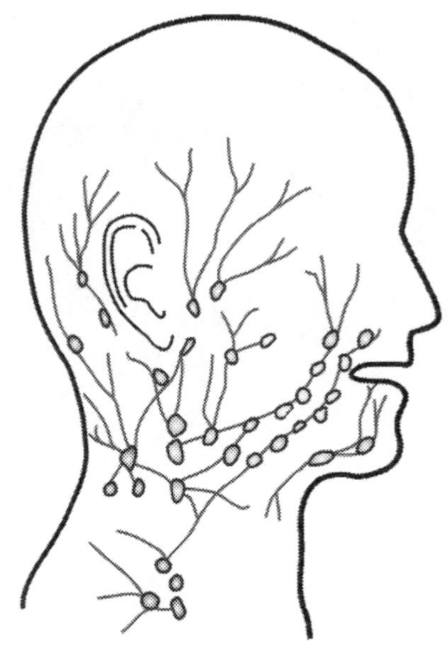

Lymph nodes in the neck area acctivated by excellent quality colostrum.

system while colostrum which contains milkings past the first milking may be less effective.

In the first milking after the cow gives birth contains 2 to 2 1/2 gallons which is 100% colostrum (of which approximately 1/2 gallon goes to the newborn calf). The second milking contains only about 20% colostrum. The rest is considered transitional milk. If this, or any other milking is mixed into the first milking, the delicate balance of colostrum components is destroyed.

Remember that researchers only use first milk colostrum of excellent quality in their trials so that if we expect to get the same beneficial results, we also need to use only first milk colostrum.

Only a small amount of excellent quality colostrum is needed to activate an immune response - just as only a light tap is needed to the first domino to set off the reaction.

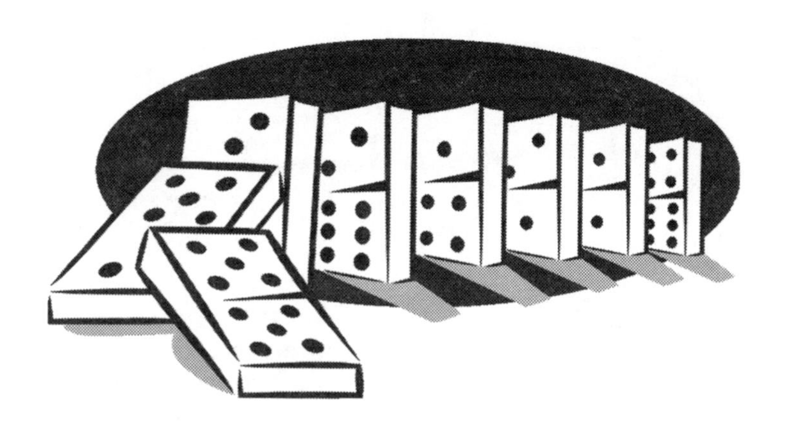

Regulation

Accessory factors

Colostrum contains peroxidase enzymes, which oxidize disease-carrying microorganisms; lactoferrin; oligosaccharides and polysaccharides, which neutralize some strains of bacteria.

Colostrum also contains immuno-regulatory factors that enhance immune reaction when it is too low and suppress it when it is too high. Colostrum therefore could be a significant tool in assisting the body in regulating the immune system. This is important for conditions in which the immune system is extremely depressed, as in severe bacterial, viral and yeast infections and in cases where the immune response is generally excessive involving inflammation and destruction (autoimmune conditions such as rheumatoid arthritis, lupus, M.S. and allergies).

Lactoferrin

Lactoferrin is the premier immuno-regulator. Lactoferrin has powerful regulating effects on the production of inflammatory cytokines. An overproduction of cytokines is commonly seen in many auto-immune conditions such as allergies, asthma, arthritis, lupus and inflammatory bowel disease. Recent research suggests that lactoferrin may be very helpful to regulate this overproduction. (Zimecki)

Lactoferrin is an iron-binding protein. Individuals with an adequate intake of iron may not be able to use the iron effectively because they may not have high enough levels of iron-binding protein to facilitate iron transport. Iron-deficient individuals experience weakness, headaches, tingling sensations in the hands and feet, brittle nails and lowered resistance to stress and disease.

Lactoferrin allows individuals to better use the iron that is in the foods they eat or in their supplements. In addition, colostrum provides essential amino acids and other nutrients in a highly desirable form. It is an excellent food source for older individuals who have compromised digestive tracts.

Proline-Rich-Polypeptides

Colostrum contains a special Proline-Rich-Polypeptide (PRP) that serves as a powerful regulator of the immune system. PRP in colostrum increases the permeability of the skin vessels, which offers a regulatory activity, stimulating or suppressing the immune response. (Staroscik)

The importance of regulating activity of the immune system is that it has the ability to stimulate or suppress the immune response. PRP is a powerful regulator of the immune system, initiating and suppressing the immune action. Suppressing the immune system is necessary to prevent the immune system from attacking the body itself, as in the case of autoimmune diseases such as rheumatoid arthritis, lupus, M.S., Alzheimer's disease and allergies. Colostrum's suppressive action may help prevent this type of activity involved in autoimmune diseases.

This component of colostrum supplementation may turn out to be even more important than we now realize. We are only in the beginning stages of realizing the total potential of PRP and other colostrum accessory factors in for the management of autoimmune/inflammatory conditions.

Support

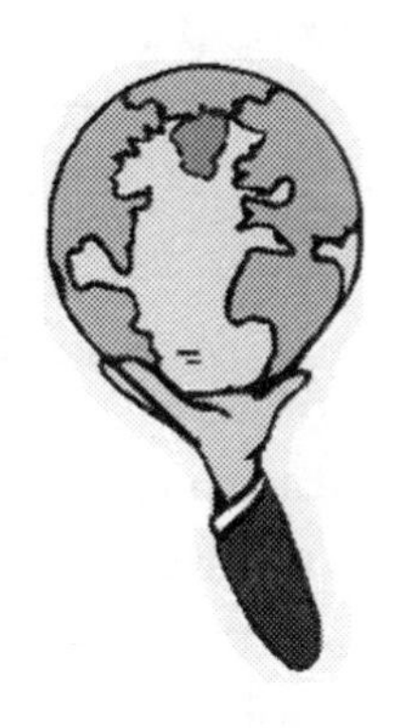

Transforming Growth Factors

Transforming Growth Factors (TGF) are polypeptides which promote cell proliferation, tissue repair and maintenance (wound healing) and embryonic development. Dr. F.J. Ballard, et al, found bovine colostrum contained up to 100 times the mitogenic potency of human colostrum. Studies have also demonstrated the anti-cancer ability of TGF in bovine colostrum in humans. (Tokuyama)

This aspect of colostrum is one which makes it especially appealing for topical use. Conditions such as eczema, dermatitis, acne, possibly psoriasis and many other other skin conditions could benefit.

Nucleotides

Nucleotides are important in cellular metabolism. The most important nucleotide in colostrum is AMP (Adenosine Monophosphate). AMP is a precursor for ADP, adenosine diphosphate, which is involved in cellular energy transfer. AMP plays a regular role in cellular metabolism and also mediates the traffic of hormones and other activators. Additional nucleotides in colostrum help metabolize carbohydrates.

Enhanced Nutrient Absorption

The elderly are at higher risk for illness and disease for a number of reasons. One is the obstacle of diminished nutrient absorption and nutrient deficiencies, which further weakens immunity. Enzymes found in colostrum help the entire digestive process to aid in nutrient absorption and utilization.

Composition of Colostrum Supplements

The composition of supplemental colostrum differs widely from one provider to another. The following information may be useful to see how extremely important excellent quality colostrum really is (quality in reference to time of collection).

QUALITY OF COLOSTRUM:	EXCELLENT	MODERATE	POOR
Total Protein:	50-60%	40-50%	<40%
Total Immunoglobulins as a % of Protein:	30-50%	20-30%	<20%
Total Fat:	13-18%	10-12%	<10%
Total Lactose:	6-11%	12-20%	>20%

Also found in trace quantities:

Vitamin A	Vitamin E	Choline
Peroxidase	Vitamin C	Vitamin D
Folic Acid	Carotinoids	Orotic Acid
Catalase	Vitamins B1, B2, B6, B12	

Colostrum For Lactose Intolerant

Lactose-intolerant individuals (regardless of body weight) can usually tolerate up to about 77 mg. lactose before a response is likely to occur. Poor quality colostrum contains higher levels of lactose compared to high quality colostrum. The sooner the collection after birth, the lower the level of lactose. The level of lactose in colostrum doubles in just 24 hours.

Unfortunately only a few companies report the level of lactose contained in their product. The following information will allow you to determine acceptable lactose levels for lactose-intolerant individuals. (Fleener)

LACTOSE INTOLERANCE

The amount of colostrum that can safely be ingested without triggering a lactose intolerance response that is based upon the quality of colostrum is:

EXCELLENT	MODERATE	POOR
700 mg.	500 mg.	350 mg.

Please note that this is not the recommended dosage of colostrum. The above amounts are merely the maximum amounts that can safely be taken by lactose-intolerant individuals at one time. Extremely good results for a variety of ailments can be achieved with as little as 125 mg. of excellent quality colostrum delivered in the oral cavity.

LACTOFERRIN

While I touched on lactoferrin as one of the regulatory components of colostrum, it is so important and has so many functions on its own that it deserves an entire section on its own.

Lactoferrin, a bioactive glycoprotein, is one of the body's own most powerful immunodefensives. While it is found in breast milk, lactoferrin is also found in small quantities in most body fluids such as saliva, tears, nasal secretions, intestinal fluids such as bile and in secondary granules of white blood cells called neutrophils. (Singleton)

It is synthesized by mucosal lining (such as in the mouth and intestinal tract) and by neutrophils, and is released by these cells in response to inflammatory stimuli. Very low physiologic serum levels of lactoferrin increase significantly upon infection. (Mann)

Receptors for lactoferrin were detected and isolated on activated T and B-cells, monocytes, intestinal brush border cells, platelets and neoplastic cells. (Adamik)

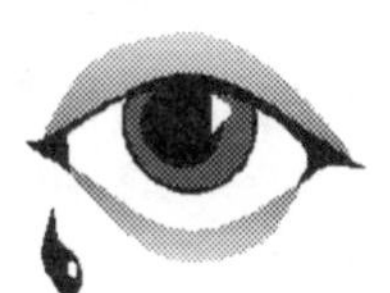

Lactoferrin is found in tears and in other body fluids located at body openings – the oral and nasal cavities, GI tract, genitourinary tract and respiratory tract. Lactoferrin is the first line of defense for any opening in the body.

The Benefits of Lactoferrin Include:

- Binds and transports iron in the body.

  - Beneficial for iron-deficiency anemia.

  - Provides unfavorable conditions for growth of certain harmful pathogens.

- Promotes intestinal cell growth (enhances nutrient digestion).

- Activates and regulates the immune system.
  - Produces or stimulates production of antibodies, interleukins, killer cells and other white blood cells, etc.

  - Enhances phagocytosis, cell adherence and controls release of proinflammatory cytokines such as IL-1, IL-6 and TNF-alpha.

- Provides unfavorable conditions for growth of certain harmful microorganisms (inhibits binding activity, etc.).

- Lactoferrin as an antioxidant diminishes the damaging effects of free radicals.

- Lactoferrin possesses interesting immunotropic properties with regard to immature T and B-cells by promoting maturation of these cells.

- Lactoferrin also controls the effector phase of cellular immune response and inhibits manifestations of autoimmune response in mice.

- One molecular form of lactoferrin with a ribonuclease activity may have value for individuals with breast cancer.

- Lactoferrin may be potentially applied in neutropenic patients or in patients with bleeding disorders as a preoperative immunomodulator. (Adamik)

Functions and Aspects of Control

Lactoferrin is closely related in structure to the plasma iron transport protein transferrin. (Singleton) The ability of lactoferrin to bind to excess iron ions, prevents the growth of bacterial and viral microorganisms and tumors, as iron is needed for their growth.

Lactoferrin also inhibits viral attack through its ability to strongly bind to the envelope protein. This prevents cell-virus fusion as the binding domain is shielded. (Swart)

Another major function of lactoferrin is its ability to stimulate the release of neutrophil-activating polypeptide interleukin 8. This suggests that lactoferrin may function as an immunomediator for activating the host defense system. Lactoferrin is implicated in particular in the control of immune functions and cell proliferation.

Researchers examining its involvement in cancer progression report that lactoferrin has a significant effect on natural killer (NK) cell cytotoxicity against certain cell lines. They also showed that lactoferrin has a normalizing effect by inhibiting cell proliferation by blocking the cell cycle progression. (Damiens)

Many other functions are attributed to lactoferrin. These include antibody synthesis, regulation and control of the production of interleukins, lymphocyte proliferation and complement activation, but the action of these functions is not fully understood.

It has been suggested that lactoferrin may contribute to T-cell proliferation. Lactoferrin regulates the iron which at low concentrations is inhibitory to T-cells. (Brock)

Lactoferrin may also have a protective function over structures such as macrophages and lymphocytes. (Brock)

Lactoferrin Regulates Inflammatory Response

One of the major benefits of lactoferrin is its ability to reduce inflammation through the regulation of inflammatory cytokines such as Interleukin-1 (IL-1, Interleukin-6 (IL-6) and tumor necrosis factor (TNF). These are a large group of chemicals largely produced by T-cells. Each one acts on a particular group of cells. While they are necessary in certain situations, too much of even a good thing can be damaging.

The problem is that high levels of these substances are seen in individuals with inflammatory autoimmune conditions such as rheumatoid arthritis, lupus, asthma, allergies, etc. The overproduction of IL-6 may explain many of the symptoms of these conditions. (Matsuda, Di Poi, Nawata, Jones)

Specifically, in individuals with rheumatoid arthritis, IL-6 is produced by the synovial fluids and contributes to inflammation, tissue damage and pain. (Matsuda)

Lactoferrin Regulates Immune Response in Critically Ill Patients

One study investigated whether lactoferrin can improve the immune competence of cells from patients with systemic inflammatory response syndrome. The researchers concluded that lactoferrin was effective in helping to regulate actions on the altered reactivity of peripheral blood mononuclear cells. Specifically, they found that lactoferrin is a good inducer of IL-6 and TNF-alpha production. (Adamik)

Lactoferrin Regulates the Immune Response in Healthy Individuals

Three groups of volunteers (7 persons per group) took one capsule containing 2, 10 or 50 mg. of bovine lactoferrin for seven days. A control group took a placebo only.

Venous blood was compared before the first dose of lactoferrin, one day and 14 days after the last dose. The following were evaluated to examine the lactoferrin effect on the immune system:

1. Content of neutrophil precursors in the peripheral blood
2. Production of IL-6
3. Production of TNF-alpha by unstimulated blood cell cultures

They found that oral treatment of lactoferrin caused an increase of newly formed neutrophils. That increase was more than 2-fold in the case of 10 mg. dose. However, significant increases in neutrophils were also registered at doses of 2 and 50 mg. of lactoferrin. No change in the neutrophil cell content was observed in the placebo group. Increased neutrophils means increased protection against invading pathogens.

The lactoferrin treatment also resulted in a beneficial effect on inflammation with the profound decrease of the spontaneous production of IL-6 and TNF-alpha. This decrease was significant (10 mg. /dose) one day following the last dose of lactoferrin and persisted for additional 14 days. (Zimecki)

Elevated IL-6 Levels in Other Conditions:

There are many more conditions with abnormal elevated IL-6 and TNF-alpha which have no published data on the effects of lactoferrin. Common sense would bring one to suspect that it may be helpful - or at least warrants further investigations. Here are two more such conditions.

Grave's Disease

Grave's Disease, also called hyperthyroidism, involves an excessive amount of thyroid hormones circulating in the blood, usually because of an over-active thyroid gland. The thyroid gland is located in the neck, below the Adam's apple. Thyroid hormones are essential for the function of every cell in the body. They help regulate growth and the rate of chemical reactions (metabolism) in the body.

Elevated levels of IL-6 are seen in individuals with Grave's Disease. (Salvi) Researchers have also shown that IL-6 levels are elevated even more so in the Grave's Disease patients with ophthalmopathy than in those without eye disease. Ophthalmopathy is an inflammatory condition that becomes more common as the Grave's Disease progresses.

One study showed elevated IL-6 levels in 22 out of 47 patients with ophthalmopathy who had thyroid disease for longer than one year in comparison with those who had it for less. The increase showed a strong association with the inflammatory signs of eye disease in the patients with Grave's compared with those without ophthalmopathy. IL-6 may be an important factor in the inflammatory events of Graves' ophthalmopathy. (Molnar)

Dr. Raymond Lombardi, Director of the Lombardi Health Center in Redding, California, reports that one of his patients who has Grave's Disease was able to decrease his thyroid medication by 1/3 after taking 4 colostrum lactoferrin lozenges per day for 3 months. The colostrum-lactoferrin lozenges were added to a comprehensive protocol of a number of other supplements, but adding the colostrum-lactoferrin lozenges is what seemed to make the difference.

Schizophrenia

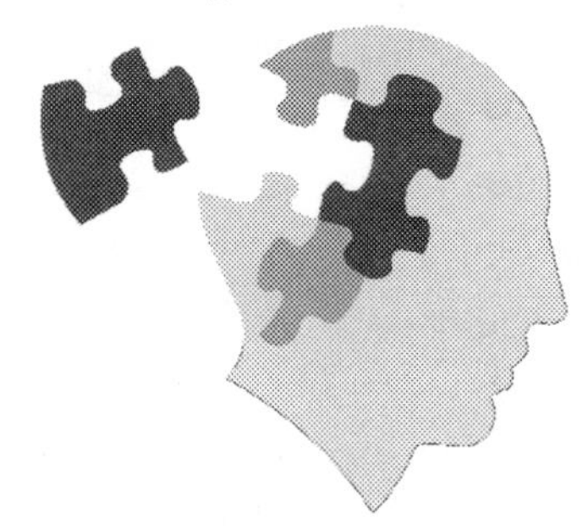

Schizophrenia is a term used to describe a complex, extremely puzzling condition, the most chronic and disabling of the major mental illnesses. Because of the disorder's complexity, few generalizations hold true for all people who are diagnosed as schizophrenic.

Elevated circulating levels of IL-6 are found in individuals with schizophrenia. Schizophrenia may result from immune or inflammatory disorders, which are mediated by cytokines.

Researchers investigated circulating levels of proinflammatory cytokines, IL-6 and TNF-alpha in serum from 30 chronic schizophrenic patients and 15 normal control. Circulating levels of IL-6 were higher in patients than in controls; those of TNF-alpha were not significantly higher than in controls. In addition, IL-6 levels were higher in patients with acute exacerbation of schizophrenia than in patients with remissions. These results suggest that immunologic abnormalities in schizophrenia may be related to a specific inflammatory process mediated by IL-6. (Naudin)

Other Benefits of Lactoferrin

Reduces Inflammation/Speeds Healing

Researchers at the Institute of Immunology and Experimental Therapy, Polish Academy of Sciences, Wroclaw, showed that bovine lactoferrin given to animals prior to surgery lowers serum IL-6 and TNF-alpha levels.

Bovine lactoferrin reduced the level of serum IL-6 70-90%, TNF-alpha by 20-30%. The data suggest that lactoferrin may find therapeutic application for diminishing manifestations of shock in inflammation caused by clinical insults. Inflammatory cytokines interfere with tissue healing. (Zimecki)

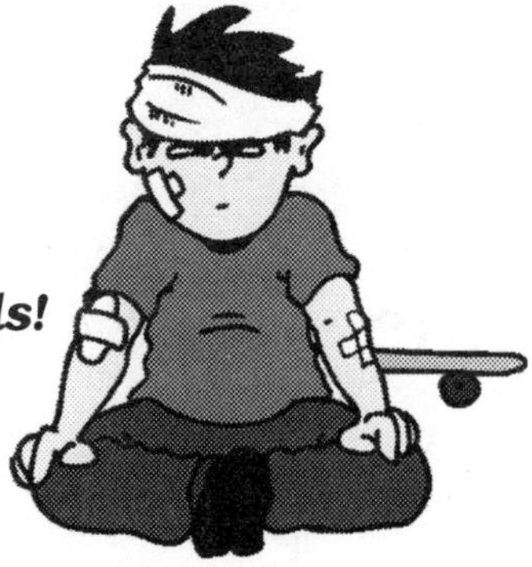

Lactoferrin can help speed healing of wounds!

Another study also conducted at the Polish Academy of Sciences on humans also showed similar benefits. Lactoferrin demonstrated an ability to reduce the proliferative response of the tissues after surgery. Reduced inflammation creates less stress and speeds healing time. Similarly, lactoferrin exhibited an inhibitory effect on IL-6 production. In low-responding patients, a considerable up-regulatory effect on TNF-alpha production, was of a special interest. The researchers suggested that lactoferrin may play a role in regulating the immune response of patients to surgery and promoting tissue regeneration. (Wlaszczyk)

Lactoferrin Has Antioxidant Effects

Lactoferrin presents differential effects in the induction of normal human monocyte activation. lactoferrin inhibits the free radical generation by normal human monocytes. (Paul-Eugene) This tissue-protecting activity would also be beneficial in inflammatory conditions such as arthritis or periodontal disease to help promote healing.

Bovine Lactoferrin More Potent than Human Lactoferrin!

Researchers in Sweden showed that the anti-inflammatory effects of bovine lactoferrin was similar to or higher than that of human lactoferrin. There studies showed addition of bovine lactoferrin caused an approximate 45% reduction of the IL-6 response. (Mattsby-Baltzer)

Both bovine and human lactoferrin provide antimicrobial activity against numerous oral pathogens. Peptides from bovine lactoferrin have been shown to have more potent antimicrobial activities than the human equivalents. (Groenink)

Bovine Lactoferrin Effective Against Hepatitis C

A pilot study conducted at the Yokohama City University School of Medicine, Japan, found that a 8-week course of bovine lactoferrin (1.8 or 3.6 grams/day) effectively prevented hepatitis C virus (HCV) infection in a significant number of individuals with chronic hepatitis C. HCV is associated with the development of cirrhosis and hepato cellular carcinoma.

Supplemental Lactoferrin

In most colostrum dietary supplements, the lactoferrin content is not sufficient unless additional amounts are supplemented. Please note that a newborn calf will ingest a half-liter or more of colostrum at its first meal and will therefore receive an adequate amount of lactoferrin. Most colostrum supplements, even at high doses of up to 2 grams per day, contain less than 2% of the lactoferrin that a newborn receives. It is far better to take the highest quality colostrum obtainable and to be sure that it is supplemented with additional lactoferrin to receive the correct balance. Lactoferrin works on contact and is therefore best utilized if taken into the oral cavity (mouth) so it can begin working right away.

COLOSTRUM-LACTOFERRIN APPLICATIONS FOR ADULTS

It is very difficult to form a complete list of all of the potential benefits of supplementing colostrum and lactoferrin. Here is a brief overview:

1. General immune enhancement - especially for immuno-compromised individuals (ill, elderly, high stress, undernourished, etc.) Helps boost resistance against illness of all kinds.

2. Antiviral/antibacterial protection–specific and non-specific

3. Protects against numerous auto-immune conditions: Arthritis, allergies, asthma, multiple sclerosis, lupus, diabetes, etc.

4. Regulation of inflammatory response

- down regulation of IL-6 and TNF inflammatory response

- boost white blood cell activity to increase resistance

5. Possible protection against development of heart disease. Lactoferrin protects cholesterol from oxidation, which damages the arteries and contributes to plaque buildup.

7. Anti-cancer protection

8. Possible lean muscle mass enhancement and faster recovery time for athletes.

9. Topical applications of colostrum and/or lactoferrin in cream form to promote wound healing from cuts, abrasions and burns, as well as minor fungal or bacterial infections, should be further investigated.

IMMUNE DEFICIENCY & SUPPRESSION

Millions of people today are in a constant state of immuno-suppression. General immune deficiency is experienced by all of us from time to time.

Immuno-suppression is largely due to stress of all kinds on the body - physical, mental and environmental. These come from nutritional deficiencies, devitalized foods, our polluted environment, exposure to pathogens, drugs (both recreational and pharmaceutical), alcohol and other external forces.

The causes of immuno-suppression are cumulative. As we are exposed to more and more stress the immune system becomes weaker and weaker. As it weakens, our ability to fight off illness decreases and the frequency of infection increases - which further weakens the immune system.

We are all provided a genetically active immune system and an acquired immune response. This means part of our immunity is inherited and the rest is obtained through accumulated responses to foreign body exposures.

The work of the immune system to fight off these stressors can gradually take its toll over the years. The effort required of the immune system varies from person to person. Genetics, sex, age and other factors come into play as well.

In general, as we get older the immune system gradually decreases in its vitality. By age 60, the immune system may be functioning at only 20% of normal capacity, especially if any of the conditions above are present.

The elderly are also faced with additional obstacles such as diminished nutrient absorption and nutrient deficiencies, which further weakens immunity. Intake of medications as well as nutrients is a grave concern for most of the elderly. Many elderly individuals pass their medications and supplements through the digestive system intact. Up to 40% of all prescription medications are not soluble in water. One solution to diminished absorption in the elderly is to introduce nutrients and medications directly into the oral cavity. Delivery of colostrum and lactoferrin directly into the mouth is not dependent upon lower GI absorption. Both of these substances in the mouth can help the entire digestive process due to the enzymes present.

On the other hand, individuals who take good care of themselves have excellent protection from their immune systems at age 60 and over.

Immune deficiency is characterized by:

- Fatigue, loss of stamina and energy
- Swollen lymph nodes
- Frequent colds and infections
- Loss of appetite and weight loss
- Fever, night sweats
- Skin rashes and cold sores
- Diarrhea, etc.

The deficient immune system is unable to effectively fight off intruders it would otherwise fight off, such as the common cold, flu, bacteria, viruses, allergens and even cancer. The degree to which we are affected depends on a number of factors, such as our general state of health and how we respond.

Colostrum and lactoferrin can be supplemented on a daily basis to enhance the immune system as a preventative against illness.

Does this mean that one will not ever get sick if using colostrum and lactoferrin? No, it does not. Most people simply report greatly enhanced immunity. For example, an individual who otherwise experienced 2-3 colds or flu per year after supplementing colostrum and lactoferrin may only experience 1 cold or flu per year. And, very importantly, instead of a recovery period of 5 to 7 days (without colostrum and lactoferrin), the recovery period may be reduced to 1-3 days when supplementing colostrum and lactoferrin.

Common Cold

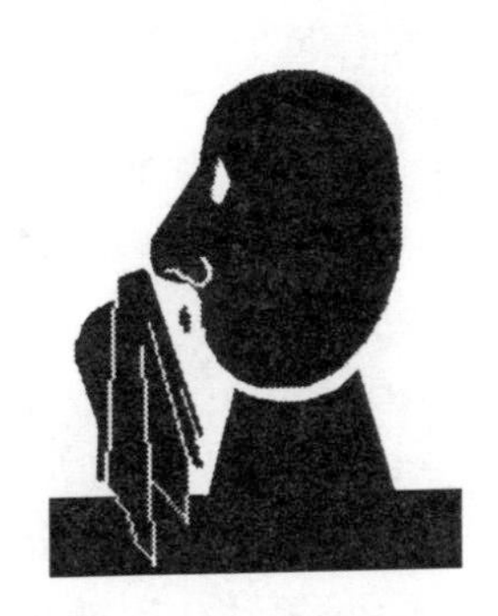

The common cold, also known as a viral upper respiratory tract infection, is a contagious illness caused by a number of different types of viruses. Because of the great number of viruses that can cause a cold, the body never builds up resistance against all of them. For this reason, colds are a frequent and recurring problem. In fact, on average, preschool children have 9 colds a year; those in kindergarten, 12 colds a year; and adolescents and adults, 7 colds per year.

Symptoms of a common cold include nasal congestion and drainage, sore throat, hoarseness, cough and perhaps a fever and headache. Many people with a cold feel tired and achy. These symptoms typically last from 3-10 days.

The common cold is spread mostly by hand-to-hand contact. For example, an infected person blows or touches his or her nose and then touches something else - telephone, computer keyboard, bathroom faucet, etc, which someone else then touches who then becomes infected with the virus. The cold virus can live on objects such as pens, books, silverware and glasses for several hours before it is picked up by someone else. While coughing and sneezing can transfer colds, they are actually poor mechanisms for spreading viruses.

Do antibiotics help the common cold?

No. Antibiotics only fight against bacterial infections, as colds are viral, antibiotics play no role in treating them. The unnecessary use of antibiotics has led to the growth of several strains of common bacte-

I came down with the worst cold I can remember having in many years. I began taking the colostrum the day I felt myself getting sick. For one day I was flat on my back and the next day I woke with just minor sniffles. Normally when I've come down with a cold like that it would take at least a week or longer to get over it. I took six or eight colostrum lozenges throughout that first day. From now on I will take them on a regular basis. I'm thoroughly impressed.

Thank you! J.G.

ria that are resistant to antibiotics (including one that commonly causes ear infections in children). For these and other reasons, it is important to limit the use of antibiotics to situations in which they are necessary.

Sometimes, an infection with bacteria can follow the cold virus. These can be treated with antibiotics.

Flu

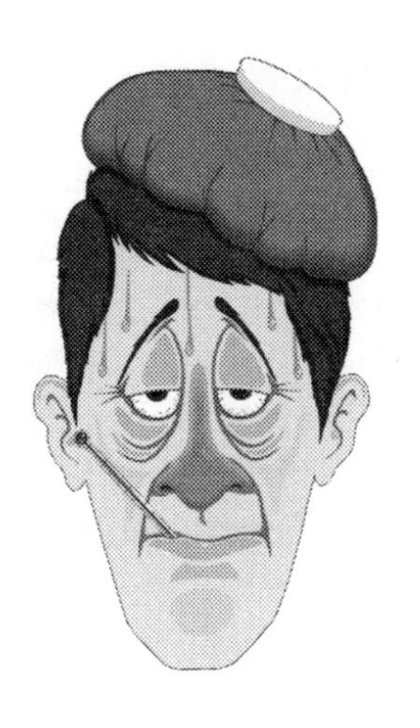

Influenza, commonly called "the flu," is caused by viruses that infect the respiratory tract. Compared with most other viral respiratory infections, such as the common cold, influenza infection often causes a more severe illness.

Influenza viruses are divided into three types, designated A, B, and C. Influenza types A and B are responsible for epidemics of respiratory illness that occur almost every winter and are often associated with increased rates of hospitalization and death. Influenza type C differs from types A and B in some important ways. Type C infection usually causes either a very mild respiratory illness or no symptoms at all; it does not cause epidemics and does not have the severe public health impact that influenza types A and B do.

Influenza viruses continually change over time, usually by mutation. This constant changing enables the virus to evade the immune system of its host, so that people are susceptible to influenza virus infection throughout life.

Most people who get the flu recover completely in 1 to 2 weeks, but some people develop serious and potentially life-threatening medical complications, such as pneumonia.

Symptoms of Influenza

Typical clinical features of influenza include fever (usually 100° F to 103° F in adults and often even higher in children) and respiratory symptoms, such as cough, sore throat, runny or stuffy nose, as well as headache, muscle aches and often extreme fatigue. Although nausea, vomiting and diarrhea can sometimes accompany influenza infection, especially in children, gastrointestinal symptoms are rarely prominent. The term "stomach flu" is a misnomer that is sometimes used to describe gastrointestinal illnesses caused by other microorganisms.

Most people who get the flu recover completely in 1 to 2 weeks, but some people develop serious and potentially life-threatening medical complications, such as pneumonia. In an average year, influenza is associated with about 20,000 deaths nationwide and many more hospitalizations. Flu-related complications can occur at any age; however, the elderly and people with chronic health problems are much more likely to develop serious complications after influenza infection than are younger, healthier people.

Colostrum For Sore Throat, Cold and Flu

In a controlled study to determine the effectiveness of colostrum on a sore throat (often one of the first signs of an oncoming cold or flu) individuals showed significant reduction of some symptoms from the first day. (Aabakken) Other related studies (against tonsillitis forming bacteria) have shown similar beneficial results. (Urban)

Why Not Strengthen and Support Our Immune System Naturally?

Every year many individuals receive flu vaccines in order to ward off infection of the flu virus. It is important to keep in mind that there are many strains of flu virus and it is impossible to create a vaccine that can prevent all of them. Vaccines are not without risk and side effects as they are created using killed or weakened viruses or bacteria. They can be very dangerous and many people suffer serious consequences. Why not strengthen your natural immunity against infection safely with colostrum and lactoferrin?

Wouldn't you rather prevent infection naturally - with colostrum and lactoferrin?

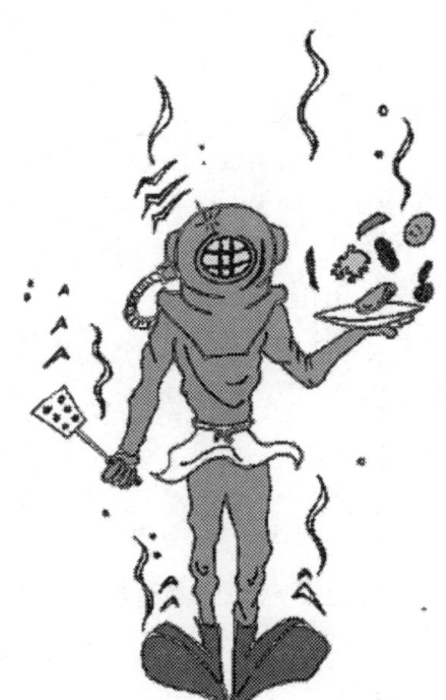

HIV and AIDS

AIDS develops as the result of the natural process of infection by the Human Immunodeficiency Virus (HIV). AIDS destroys the body's immune system and allows otherwise controllable infections to invade the body and cause additional diseases. These unusual infections and cancers are not a threat to individuals with healthy immune systems.

These "opportunistic" infections, Pneumocystis Carinli Pneumonia (PCP), Kaposi's Sarcoma (KS), severe yeast infections (candidiasis), viral infections (herpes and cytomegalovirus), parasitic infections (Cryptosporidium parvum), and unusual lymphomas which would not otherwise gain a foothold in the body, may eventually cause death.

HIV may also attack the nervous system and cause delayed damage to the brain. This damage may take years to develop and the symptoms may show up as memory loss, indifference, loss of coordination, partial paralysis or mental disorder. Any of these symptoms may occur alone, or concurrent with other symptoms mentioned earlier.

HIV is spread through the exchange of blood and body fluid, largely by sexual contact with an infected partner through small lacerations in the body's mucosa lining (for example, small tears in the vagina or rectum), or sharing needles with an infected intravenous drug user. Infected pregnant women may transmit the virus to their babies.

While transfusion of contaminated blood is a mode of transmission, since 1985 all blood donated in blood banks is tested for the presence of antibody to HIV.

HIV and the Immune System

When HIV enters the bloodstream it attaches to a host cell and installs its genetic material. It simply moves in and takes over!

The virus can then make thousands of copies of itself in a very short time. HIV seems to prefer certain cells in the immune system as host cells: macrophages and T-helper cells. These two types of immune cells normally interact together against intruders to defend the body.

HIV destroys this defense system by attacking T-helper cells, infiltrating macrophages and disrupting the normal communication between the two. T-helper cells, which normally are responsible for initiating immune responses, cannot alert the remainder of the immune system to the presence of HIV.

The decrease in T-helper cells seems to increase the number of T-suppressor cells. T-suppressor cells normally tell the immune system to shut off because the enemy is under control. This leaves the body unable to defend itself against illnesses ranging from the common cold to KS and PCP, which may otherwise be combatted effectively.

Macrophages, unlike T-helper cells which are killed, seem to tolerate HIV infection. In the macrophage, HIV "hides" in small pockets called vacuoles inside the cell where the immune system cannot see it. The virus can thrive there, safe from attack. A stimulus, such as infection by a herpes virus, might then send the HIV into high reproductive gear causing new viruses to escape from the host.

Macrophages infected with HIV can also pass on the infection to other cells by just touching them.

Substances released by infected macrophages damage brain cells. This may be the reason half of all AIDS patients develop neurological problems.

There still is no cure for AIDS. In 1996, Merck and Co, Inc. introduced the protease inhibitor drug (Crixovan® – generic name, Indinavir-Sulfate). When used in conjunction with other drugs such as AZT (generic name, Zidivudine) and Epivir (generic name, Lamnivudine), they have proven to stop HIV replication in the blood stream and reduce the viral load in HIV-positive individuals. Many cases report that the virus is no longer detectable in the blood. The virus is believed to still be present in lymph and brain tissues so the therapy is not yet deemed a cure, but it is certainly good news. Individuals taking these medications are experiencing a rise in T-cells and an improved immune system.

An undetectable viral load also does not mean that there is no risk of transmission of the virus to others. There is still the possibility of infecting others.

Lactoferrin Inhibits HIV

A number of native and modified milk proteins from bovine or human sources were analyzed for their inhibitory effects on HIV-1 and HIV-2 in vitro. The proteins investigated were lactoferrin, alpha-lactalbumin, beta-lactoglobulin A, and beta-lactoglobulin B. They all showed a strong antiviral activity against HIV-1 and/or 2.

All compounds showed virtually no cytotoxicity at the concentrations used. The antiviral action was believed to be caused by the inhibition of virus-cell fusion and entry of the virus into MT4 cells. (Swart)

In another study, proteins purified from serum

and milk were assayed to assess their inhibiting capacity on HIV and human cytomegalovirus (HCMV) on MT4 cells and fibroblasts, respectively. Lactoferrin also inhibited the HIV-induced cytopathic effect. When negatively charged groups were added to lacto-ferrin, there was a four-fold stronger antiviral effect on HIV, but the antiviral potency for HCMV infection was mostly decreased. Lactoferrin either reduces viral absorption or penetration or both. (Harmsen)

Researchers in Rome at the Laboratory of Immunology, Istituto Superioredi Sanita, reported that bovine lactoferrin had potent antiviral activity against HIV. They found that both HIV-1 replication and syncytium formation were efficiently inhibited, in a dose-dependent manner by lactoferrins. Bovine lactoferrin markedly inhibited HIV-1 replication when added prior to HIV infection or during the virus adsorption step, thus suggesting a mechanism of action on the HIV binding to or entry into C8166 cells (a type of T-cell typically attacked by HIV). (Puddu)

Lactoferrin Levels Low in Individuals with HIV

Levels of plasma lactoferrin are decreased in HIV-infected patients in relation to the progression of the disease. Plasma lactoferrin concentrations were determined using a specific and sensitive enzyme immunoassay. Ninety-seven subjects were studied (22 asymptomatic and 45 symptomatic patients compared to 30 healthy controls). The results showed a highly significant decrease in the level of lactoferrin in HIV-infected patients compared to controls.

The plasma for symptomatic patients showed their average lactoferrin level at 0.36 mcg./ml., still far above the normal values. In view of the important biological effects of lactoferrin, the lack of such a molecule could be one important component of the nature of HIV infection.

The analysis of a group of late stage AIDS patients showed a decrease in lactoferrin produced by the oral mucosa in comparison with HIV-negative controls. This was associated with an increase in albumin, which indicates an alteration of the mucosal barrier. (Lu)

Colostrum for Candida/Mouth Sores

Oral candidiasis is common among HIV positive individuals. Lactoferrin, lysozyme, secretory IgA and numerous other important protective factors in a colostrum lozenge can offer excellent localized (and systemic) immune protective benefits to individuals with compromised mucosal immunity.

In the late 1980's, researchers from Denmark reported at the European Conference on Clinical Aspects of HIV Infection in Brussels that colostrum tablets proved to be effective treatment for thrush (oral candida) among HIV-infected individuals, given ten times a day for ten days. (Christensen)

A well-known Finnish researcher, A. Lassus, M.D., also reported that as colostrum acts as a natural antibiotic, that it is effective for painful ulcers in the mouth. A colostrum lozenge (containing 60 mg. immunoglobulins), 10 times a day for seven days encouraged spontaneous healing in a placebo-controlled study. The healing time was shortened and pain was diminished in the first day in some patients. (Lassus)

	AVERAGE HEALING TIME	AVERAGE DURATION OF PAIN
Active Treatment	3 days	6.9 days
Placebo Treatment	1.7 days	5.3 days

Colostrum Stops Diarrhea Caused by C. Parvum

Cryptosporidium Parvum (C. parvum) is an opportunistic parasite infection common among individuals with HIV. It is the most common cause of the frequently experienced diarrhea. The parasite robs nutrients and energy from the infected person causing rapid weight loss and malnutrition, which further weakens the immune system.

Diarrhea and weight loss are found in more than 50% of patients with AIDS. The symptoms can be very severe, leading to death even in the absence of opportunistic infections. In 30% of these patients, the pathogens cannot be identified, and approximately only half of the identifiable etiologic agents of diarrhea in HIV patients are treatable with antibiotics.

Immunoglobulins from bovine colostrum contain high levels of antibodies against a wide range of bacterial, viral and protozoal pathogens as well as against various bacterial toxins. It is quite resistant to 24-hour incubation with gastric juice (they are not broken down in the stomach and therefore able to provide protective benefits).

In a multi-center pilot study, 37 immunodeficient patients with chronic diarrhea were treated with oral bovine colostrum immunoglobulins (10 g./day for 10 days). Good therapeutic effects were observed. Out of

31 treatment periods in 29 HIV-infected patients, 21 gave good results leading to transient (10 days) or long-lasting (more than four weeks) normalization of the stool frequency. The mean daily stool frequency decreased from 7.4 to 2.2 at the end of the treatment. Eight HIV-infected patients showed no response. The diarrhea recurred in 12 patients within four weeks (32.4%), while 19 patients were free of diarrhea for at least four weeks (51.3%). In five patients, intestinal C. parvum disappeared. Bovine colostrum immunoglobulins treatment was also beneficial in 4 out of 5 graft versus host disease patients. (Rump)

A number of additional clinical studies have also shown that colostrum is very beneficial in treating individuals infected with C. parvum diarrhea. Supplementing dried colostrum promoted weight gain and restored energy. (Nord)

In a study of 24 patients with severe chronic diarrhea and AIDS, patients were stratified to one of three cohorts: (1) C. parvum infection alone, (2) C. parvum and a second opportunistic infection, and (3) idiopathic AIDS enteropathy with no identified source of infection or an untreatable opportunistic infection other than C. parvum. All patients were treated with bovine immunoglobulin concentrate for 21 days.

The primary benefit was the decrease in daily stool weight. Additional benefits included decrease in stool frequency and improved body weight, as well as clearance of C. parvum oocytes (eggs).

Patients with C. parvum who were treated with bovine immunoglobulin concentrate in powder form experienced a significant decrease in mean stool weight one month after completing treatment. The stool frequency decreased during the treatment. Patients who received bovine immunoglobulin concentrate in capsule form and patients without C. parvum (cohort 3) showed no improvement. No serious side effects were observed, and it was well tolerated. The optimal dosage, duration of therapy and overall efficacy need to be determined in placebo-controlled trials. (Greenberg)

In a study with 25 HIV patients with chronic diarrhea and either c. parvum or absence of demonstrable pathogenic organisms were treated with a daily oral dose of 10 grams of a bovine colostrum immunoglobulin preparation for 10 days. Among the seven patients with C. parvum, this treatment led to complete remission in three and partial remission in two. Among the 18 patients with diarrhea and negative stool culture, seven obtained complete remission of diarrhea and four obtained partial remission.

In the remaining two patients with C. parvum and the seven patients with diarrhea but no demonstrable pathogens, the treatment produced no significant improvement. Subsequent doubling of the dose (2 x 10 grams daily) in eight of the nonresponders led to complete remission in one case and at least partial remission in an additional four patients. The researchers concluded that treatment of diarrhea with 10 grams immunoglobulins from bovine colostrum per day constitutes an important therapeutic approach and led to complete (40%) or partial (24%) remission of diarrhea in 64% of the patients. (Plettenberg)

Cancer

Cancer is the abnormal growth of cells in our bodies. Cancer originates as a result of normal cell mutation through its genetic chromosome material, RNA and DNA. Normally, cells replicate themselves continually at a rate synchronous with normal growth and repair in a manner specific for its purpose in the body. A cancerous cell multiplies faster than it should and loses normal differentiation.

The actual mechanisms by which cancer is caused is still speculative. Quite simply, it involves a breakdown of the immune system. At any given time, there are literally thousands of "precancerous" mutated cells throughout the body. A healthy immune system is able to effectively locate and eliminate them from the body. If it does not, the mutated cells turn into cancer.

The best way to avoid cancer is to avoid known carcinogens - exessive sun exposure, tobacco, alcohol, nitrates, artificial sweeteners, pesticides and other chemicals, etc.

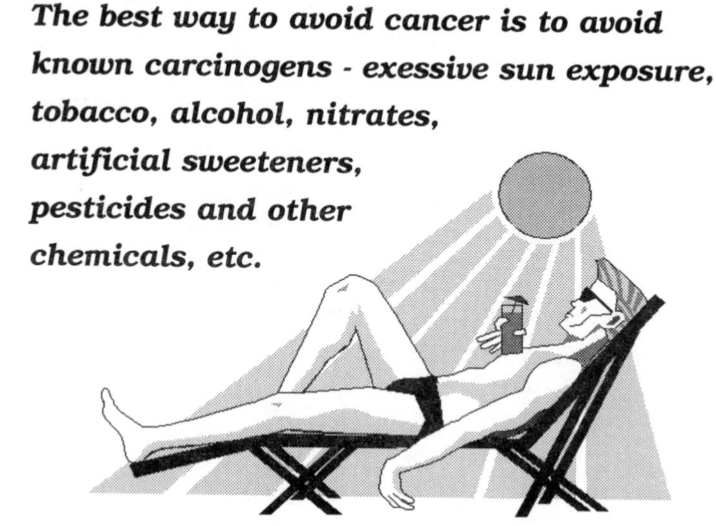

We have all heard that cancer prevention is the best way to fight cancer. We are told not to smoke or drink and to avoid foods containing nitrates, pesticides, chemicals, stress and the sun (at least without sun- screen). These are all good suggestions, but the hidden message is that these things weaken our most important defense against cancer- the immune system.

What is better than colostrum and lactoferrin to activate, regulate and balance the immune system?

Maintaining a healthy intracellular environment helps prevent cancer, and correcting a toxic environment may lead to successful non-toxic treatment for cancer. Colostrum contains powerful protective agents such as lactoferrin, interferon, transforming growth factors, PRP, enzymes and more.

Transforming Growth Factors in Colostrum Inhibit Cancer Cell Growth

Japanese researchers showed that transforming growth factor-beta-like peptides in bovine colostrum inhibited the growth of cancer cells. The investigation showed that TGF-beta-like peptide purified from bovine colostrum, remarkably suppressed growth of cancer cells. The researchers also noted an intriguingly striking change in cancer size. (Tokuyama)

Colostrum Inhibits Lymphoma, Bone Cancer and Other Cancer Types

Researchers investigating the effect of human colostrum on T-cell immune function found that colostrum inhibited the proliferation of human T-cells through inhibition of the production of IL-2 by Con A-activated human peripheral blood T-cells and by Con A-activated Jurkat cells, a human T-lymphoma line. Human colostrum also inhibited the production of IL-2 by EL-4 cells, a murine thymoma line (usually a benign tumor of the thymus associated with immune deficiency). The inhibitory activity was not toxic, and was free of side effects. (Hooton)

A Finnish study demonstrated that a medium based on bovine colostrum and adult bovine serum can be used successfully as a fetal bovine serum substitute in the culture of several anchorage-dependent and independent cell lines, including a type of bone cancer and mouse mammary tumor cell line. (Viander)

Lactoferrin Possesses Anti-tumor Effects

Lactoferrin also reduces the damaging effects of free radicals, known cancer risk factors. Lactoferrin promotes other immune activities in the body by promoting maturation of immature T- and B-cells. One molecular form of lactoferrin with a ribonuclease activity may have value against breast cancer. (Adamik)

Researchers examining its involvement in cancer progression report that lactoferrin has a significant effect on enhancing natural killer (NK) cell ability to attack haematopoietic and breast epithelial cell lines. The study also demonstrated that lactoferrin inhibits epithelial cell proliferation by blocking the cell cycle progression. (Damiens)

It will be interesting to see if topical use of colostrum and lactoferrin have any protective affects against skin cancer. No research has been conducted yet that I am aware of.

Lactoferrin Inhibits Tumor Growth

Researchers have demonstrated that lactoferrin inhibited tumor growth in mice of transplantable solid tumors. Lactoferrin also substantially reduced lung colonization by melanoma cells in mice. Iron-saturated and apo-lactoferrin exhibited comparable levels of tumor inhibition and antimetastatic activity. The researchers claimed the results for lactoferrin suggest a potentially important role for this molecule in the primary defense against tumor growth and formation. (Bezault)

Some interesting research has been conducted in this area as lactoferrin is known to bind to macrophages/monocytes and intestinal mucosal cells. Researchers examined the interaction of lactoferrin with mononuclear and colon cancer cells. They found that the cells bound more lactoferrin than transferrin. Lactoferrin significantly reduced uptake of non-transferrin-bound iron by the cells. Thus lactoferrin, unlike transferrin, is not an important iron donor to monocytic cells, but may instead serve to regulate iron uptake from other sources. It did not seem to enhance iron transport across mucosal cells. (Brock)

Much more work needs to be done in this area to determine the full cancer-protective potential of colostrum and lactoferrin.

Since 1985 cytokines found in colostrum (interleukins 1-6 and 10, interferon G, and lymphokines) have been one of the most researched protocols in scientific research for the cure of cancer. Also, colostrum lactalbumin has been found to be able to create the selective death (apoptosis) of cancer cells, leaving the surrounding noncancerous tissues unaffected.

The mixture of immune and growth factors in colostrum can inhibit the spread of cancer cells. If viruses are involved in either the intiation or the spread of cancer, colostrum could prove to be one of the best ways to prevent and control the disease.

For all of the above factors, I strongly recommend cancer patients to include colostrum in their fight against cancer.

In addition, for cancer chemotherapy patients, colostrum lessens adverse effects of cytotoxic agents. It actually enhances chemotherapy so people can take greater dosages without getting so deathly sick.

Kenneth D. Johnson, S.M.D., S.N.D., O.M.D., Ph.D., International Orthomolecular Nutritionist

Chronic Fatigue Syndrome

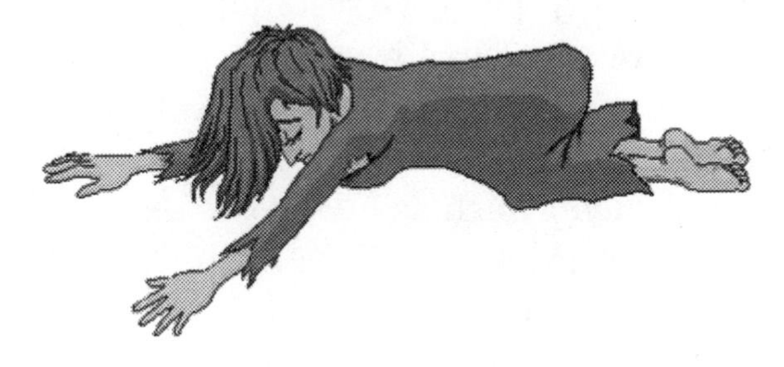

Chronic Fatigue Syndrome (CFS) is believed to be caused by the Epstein-Barr Virus (EBV), the same virus that causes mononucleosis. EBV is a member of the herpes family and is related to the viruses that cause genital herpes and shingles. Many people can carry the virus and therefore, pass it on because it is highly contagious, but have no symptoms.

Chronic Fatigue is characterized by extreme weakness and exhaustion, persistent apathy and depression, memory loss, headache, impaired concentration, recurrent achiness, low-grade fever, swollen glands, digestive problems, exaggerated allergic reactions and aggravation of preexisting conditions. Candida albicans infection is also often found in conjunction with EBV.

The condition is three times more common in women than in men. Antibodies for EBV can be detected to determine if this is the cause of the many symptoms which can last for six months or longer. There is no drug cure for EBV. It may go in remission, but if the immune system is stressed, it will begin replicating again, causing symptoms to return.

The virus causes an over-reaction of the immune system. The immune system becomes so overburdened the result is immunity "burnout." The result is a feeling of complete exhaustion. Individuals with EBV require a comprehensive restorative program for the immune system. This involves not only eliminating immunosuppressive items (sugar, caffeine, alcohol, tobacco, processed refined foods, etc.) but supportive supplements such as high doses of vitamin C, CoQ10, probiotics, vitamins A and E, etc. And what is better than colostrum and lactoferrin to activate, regulate and balance the immune system?

I am 22 years old and was diagnosed with Chronic Fatigue Syndrome in late 1998. I was experiencing migraine headaches, digestive problems. frequent illnesses and infections, required up to 12 hours sleep at night and was too tired to exercise.

After only days of taking colostrum-lactoferrin lozenges my headaches were gone, my digestive problems were greatly reduced and I am sleeping much better and can exercise almost daily without difficulty. My immune system was greatly strengthened as I have not gotten sick - not even a sore throat- in spite of all the illnesses circulating around me.

After several weeks I stopped taking the lozenges and soon many of the difficulties associated with CFS returned. Now I am afraid to not take at least one lozenge per day.

Thank you! S.W.

Colostrum-Lactoferrin Inhibit Herpes Activity

There are also a number of studies showing that colostrum and lactoferrin inhibit the replication of several strains of herpes viruses, including Herpes Simplex type 1 and 2 (Marchetti, Siciliano, Hasegawa). Lactoferrin is also known to prevent virus absorption and/or penetration into host cells, indicating an effect on the early events of virus infection. The researchers state that lactoferrin possesses a potent antiviral activity and may be useful in preventing certain herpes viral infection in humans. (Hasegawa)

Studies also indicate that individuals with acute viral infections have reduced lactoferrin content as compared with normal. This suggests an acquired defect of neutrophil lactoferrin synthesis in viral infection. (Baynes)

Hopefully, there will soon be human clinical trials to demonstrate the effect of colostrum and lactoferrin on EBV. Meanwhile, people with Chronic Fatigue Syndrome continue to report the good results they have been experiencing.

In my experience, the patients who gain the most from colsotrum-lactoferrin are those with compromised immunity, chronic and recurrent disease symptoms such as chronic fatigue syndrome, Crohn's disease, infectious diarrhea, sinusitis, and fibromyalgia.

Kenneth D. Johnson, S.M.D., S.N.D., O.M.D., Ph.D., International Orthomolecular Nutritionist

Therapeutic Recommendations for Immuno-compromised Individuals

Excellent quality colostrum liquid can be effectively used for severely immuno-compromised individuals. Therapeutic doses of an excellent quality colostrum liquid are as follows:

First 10 days: 1 Tablespoon 3 times per day

Next 10 days: 1 Tablespoon 2 times per day

Next 30 days: 1 Tablespoon 1 time per day/reevaluate

The above regime is for excellent quality colostrum liquid only. Moderate or poor quality colostrum may require more and will have unpredictable results.

The fat and casein are removed in liquid colostrum. As a result, the levels of some of the components, such as PRP, are of a higher concentration. This important, powerful regulatory Proline-Rich-Polypeptide is very important for individuals with debilitating conditions.

While the many important effects of PRP are beyond the scope of this book, I do however, want to point out one very interesting Polish study I came across on Alzheimer's Disease.

In a 12-month, double-blind trial with a PRP complex isolated from colostrum (orally delivered), 8 of 15 Alzheimer's patients improved. In the 7 others the disease stabilized. In contrast, none of the 31 patients receiving selenium or a placebo with similar mild or moderate Alzheimer's improved. The results obtained showed that PRP improves the outcome of Alzheimer's patients with mild to moderate dementia. (Leszek)

AUTOIMMUNE DISEASES

At the heart of the immune system is the ability to distinguish between self and nonself. Virtually every body cell carries distinctive molecules that identify it as self.

Sometimes the immune system's recognition apparatus breaks down, and the body begins to manufacture antibodies and T-cells directed against its own cells, cell components, or specific organs. Such antibodies are known as autoantibodies, and the conditions that result are called autoimmune diseases. (Not all autoantibodies are harmful; some types appear to be integral to the immune system's regulatory scheme.)

Autoimmune diseases affect the immune system at several levels. In patients with (Systemic Lupus Erythematosus or SLE), for instance, some aspects of the immune system are hyperactive while other parts are underactive. Also seen is a defective suppressor

Some autoimmune conditions such as rheumatoid arthritis, can be debilitating.

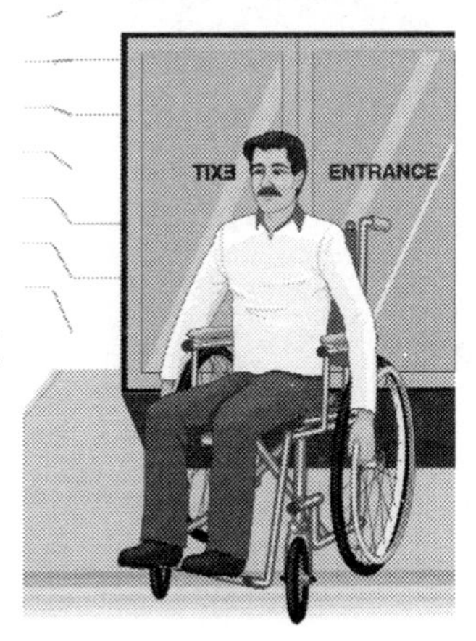

T-cell system which continues to make antibodies to a common virus, where normally the response would shut down after 10 or 12 days.

Autoimmunity contributes to many different conditions. For instance, autoantibodies to red blood cells can cause anemia, autoantibodies to pancreas cells contribute to juvenile diabetes and autoantibodies to nerve and muscle cells causing chronic muscle weakness is known as myasthenia gravis. An autoantibody known as rheumatoid factor is common in persons with rheumatoid arthritis. In some people, an apparently harmless substance such as ragweed pollen or cat hair can provoke the immune system to set off the inappropriate and harmful response known as an allergic reaction.

The following are recognized as autoimmune conditions:

Allergies

Asthma

Systemic Lupus Erythematosus (SLE)

Multiple Sclerosis (MS)

Myasthenia Gravis

Rheumatoid Arthritis

Chronic Lymphocytic Thyroiditis

Ulcerative Colitis (discussed later in the chapter concerning digestive disorders)

No one knows just what causes an autoimmune disease, but several factors are likely to be involved. These may include viruses and environmental factors such as exposure to sunlight, certain chemicals and some drugs, which may damage or alter body cells so that they are no longer recognizable as self. Sex hormones may be important, too, since most autoimmune diseases are far more common in women than in men. Heredity also appears to play a role.

In conditions established as autoimmune diseases, treatment includes anti-inflammatory and drugs that suppress the production of antibodies. This immune suppression often leads to other complications and increases risk of infection and illness.

Allergies

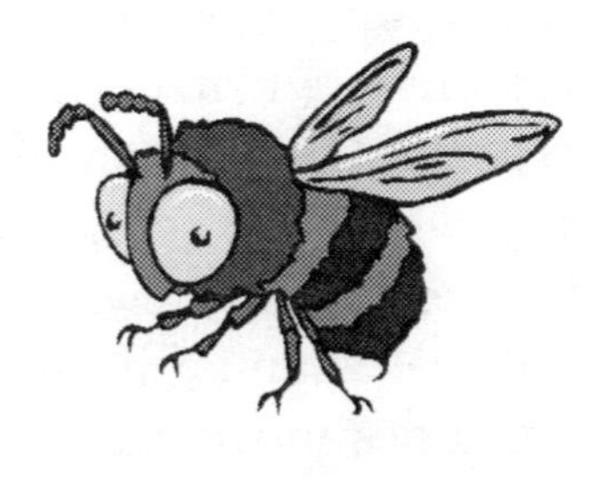

An allergy is a sensitivity to some particular otherwise inert substance known as an allergen. An allergen can be a food, an inhalant such as pollen, mold, dust, animal dander or hair, an insect sting, chemicals as well as a number of additional types.

An allergic reaction may manifest as hay fever (watery eyes, runny nose, sinus congestion, etc.), asthma, hives, eczema, high blood pressure, abnormal fatigue, abnormal hunger, stomach cramps, vomiting, anxiety, depression and other mental disorders, constipation, stomach ulcers, dizziness, headache, hyperactivity, insomnia, hypoglycemia, etc.

Susceptibility to an allergen depends on heredity and the condition of one's immune system. Stress and hypoglycemia (adrenal exhaustion), poor diet (vitamins C and B Complex deficiency), high copper levels, inadequate sleep, poor eliminations, emotional trauma and infection can weaken the immune system making one more susceptible to an allergic reaction. Colostrum can help boost one's overall immunity and decrease inflammation.

An allergic reaction frequently involves symptoms that involve inflammation: Puffed, watery eyes, sinusitis, asthma, eczema, hives, contact dermatitis, even very dangerous anaphylactic reactions where the tongue or throat swells.

Inflammation can become more manageable with the regulating factors (PRP) in colostrum, which lowers one's sensitivity point, suppressing the immune reaction. Lactoferrin helps reduce inflammatory factors which can reduce the severity of reactions.

Research shows that individuals with hayfever (allergic rhinitis) have higher levels of inflammatory cytokines in the nasal mucosa compared to controls. (Saito) Lactoferrin helps regulate and reduce these inflammatory factors, which can reduce the onset of problems.

As pointed out earlier, infants who are breast-fed have a lower frequency of allergic, inflammatory and autoimmune diseases and lymphomas in their later life when compared with that observed in children who have been formula-fed after birth. (Vassilev) Adults may also benefit from the same factors offering this protection. The self-reacting autoantibodies in colostrum serum play a major role in the selection of the pre-immune B-cell repertoire and in the maintenance of the immune homeostasis.

Asthma

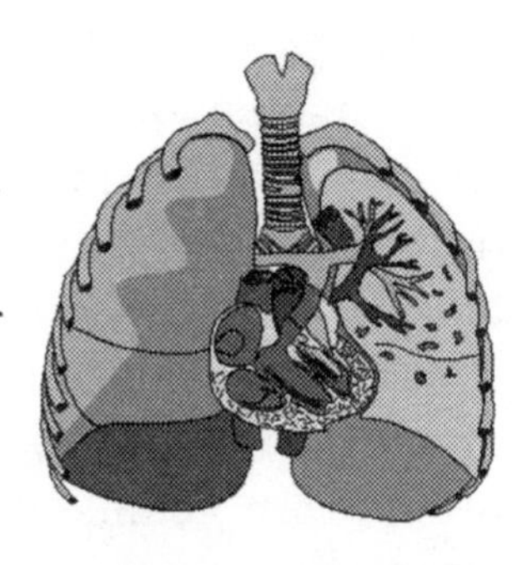

Asthma is a respiratory condition that prevents free breathing due to a number of conditions. The bronchial airways become constricted preventing normal airflow. The asthmatic's lungs are super-sensitive and easily provoked into constriction. Reactions may be triggered by dust, cat dander, pollen, cigarette smoke, perfume, a freshly mowed lawn, exercise, cold air, stress or even laughing.

Constricted airways mean that it takes great effort to force the air through. This creates a wheezing sound. Coughing is another common symptom of asthma triggered by excess mucus irritating the passages.

Most of the super-sensitivity problems of asthma, in a large number of people, are inflammation related. The inflammation is a defensive reaction of the bronchials against the allergen or irritant. Once irritated, inflammation in the lung is initiated and it tends to remain in a hypersensitive inflammatory state. This is why steroids and steroid inhalers tend to be the drug of choice by most physicians treating asthma. Steroid inhalers work by blocking the inflammatory component directly in the lung.

The PRP in colostrum helps regulate or lower the sensitivity point of the lungs, suppressing the immune action. Colostrum forces the differentiation of certain cells so that the lungs are less sensitive. The initial reaction may still occur, but far less severely, making the asthma much more manageable.

Studies show that concentrations of IL-6 and TNF-alpha are much higher in asthamatics than in controls. (Subratty) Lactoferrin helps regulate and reduce these inflammatory factors, which can reduce the severity of reactions and possibly reduce the onset of attacks. Anti-inflammatory drugs, such as prednisone, are commonly prescribed to asthmatics for this same purpose.

Lactoferrin Diminishes Bronchial Constriction

Recent biological and immunological investigations have implicated tryptase, which is an enzyme release from mast cells, as a cause of numerous allergic and inflammatory conditions including rhinitis, conjunctivitis and most notably, asthma. Tryptase is also implicated in certain gastrointestinal, dermatological and cardiovascular disorders. (Rice)

Lactoferrin may play a regulatory role as it inhibits tryptase activity. (Cregar) The physiological function of neutrophil lactoferrin may be the inhibition of tryptase released from mast cells tryptase involvement in both late-phase bronchoconstriction and airway hyperreactivity. (Elrod)

One interesting study examined the effects of lactoferrin in allergic sheep on asthma. The study showed that lactoferrin inhibits tryptase, a potential causative agent of bronchial spasm that is released by activated mast cells (such as by an antigen or irritant). (Cregar) Aerosolized lactoferrin (10 mg. in 3 ml. buffered saline solution) was given 1/2 hour prior to as well as 4 and 24 hours after they were exposed to an inhalation challenge. The lactoferrin diminished the bronchial constriction and airway hyperresponsiveness 4 and 24 hours after exposure to an antigen. (Elrod)

It would be interesting to see additional studies on humans to see what benefits of supplemental lactoferrin are available to asthmatics.

Lupus

Lupus (Systemic Lupus Erythematosus or SLE) is a chronic inflammatory autoimmune condition. Patients with lupus have unusual antibodies in their blood that target their own body cells and tissues.

B-cells are hyperactive while suppressor cells are underactive, production of IL-2 is low, while levels of gamma interferon are high.

Lupus can cause disease of the skin, heart, lungs, kidneys, joints and nervous system. When only the skin is involved, the condition is called Discoid Lupus. When internal organs are involved, the condition is called Systemic Lupus Erythematosus (SLE).

Persons with SLE, whose symptoms encompass many systems, have antibodies to many types of cells and cellular components. These include antibodies directed against substances found in the cell's genetic material. These antibodies can cause serious damage when they link up with self antigens to form circulating immune complexes, which become lodged in body tissue and set off inflammatory reactions.

Lupus is about eight times more common in women than men. The disease can affect all ages, but most commonly begins from age 20 to 45 years. It is more frequent in people of African-American, Chinese and Japanese descent.

IL-6 and TNF-alpha Levels Elevated in Lupus

Cytokine production of IL-6 and TNF-alpha is elevated in whole blood cell cultures of patients with SLE. (Swaak) Another study showed that the presence of the inflammatory cytokines IL-6 and TNF-alpha in kidneys of patients with Lupus Nephritis as an indicator of their possible role in its pathogenesis. Inflammatory cytokines are actively synthesized in the kidneys of patients with Lupus Nephritis and believed by the researchers to be in part responsible for problems associated with the condition. (Herrera-Esparza)

Because lactoferrin helps normalize production of both IL-6 and TNF-alpha, individuals with lupus may benefit greatly. Most evidence so far is anecdotal. Hopefully, clinical trials will soon demonstrate it's full

A woman with SLE in Manchester, U.K., reports she is happily able to breast-feed her newborn. Women with lupus commonly experience complications following child birth and are placed on medication (such as methotrexate) and are unable to breast-feed. She has been supplementing colostrum and a vitamin and mineral formulation. She contributed her current excellent status to the colostrum. (D.C.)

potential. Colostrum and lactoferrin may also help support the immune system in general as individuals with lupus are at high risk for a variety of other health problems including periodontal disease, frequent colds and flu, etc.

Multiple Sclerosis (MS)

Multiple sclerosis (MS) is a chronic inflammatory disease of the central nervous system, the nerves that comprise the brain and spinal cord. It is characterized by focal T-cells and macrophage infiltrates that lead to degeneration of the myelin (the fatty protective covering of nerve fibers) and loss of neurologic function. It is referred to as an autoimmune condition because the immune system treats the myelin sheath as though it were foreign, gradually destroying it and causing subsequent scarring and damage to some of the underlying nerve fibers.

In some, optic neuritis, the inflammation of the nerves in the eye, is the first symptom of MS. Vision, usually in one eye, becomes unclear or doubled, and there may be a shimmering effect. Pain, involuntary jerking or movement of the eye may also occur.

The general theory for the development of MS is that a genetically damaged immune system is unable to distinguish between virus proteins and the body's own myelin and produces antibodies that attack. In other words, the body becomes allergic to itself, a condition known as autoimmunity.

The true cause of MS in unknown and neither a

cure nor safe and effective treatments have been able to halt its progression to date.

Does a Virus Trigger MS?

Previous virological and immunological studies have suggested that MS may be triggered by a viral infection. In order to inhibit the growth of the measles virus in the patient, researchers obtained an IgA-rich cow colostrum containing antimeasles lactoglobulin resistant to proteases. This colostrum was orally administered to patients with MS to investigate its effect. Measles-positive antibody colostrum was orally administered every morning to 15 patients with MS at a daily dosage of 100 ml. for 30 days. Similarly, measles-negative antibody control colostrum was orally administered to five patients. As a clinical assessment, disability scores developed by the International Federation of Multiple Sclerosis Societies were used.

As a result of seven high level anti-measles colostrum recipients, five patients improved and two remained unchanged. Among eight low level anti-measles colostrum recipients, five patients improved and three remained unchanged.

However, of five negative colostrum recipients two patients remained unchanged and three worsened. No side effects were observed in colostrum recipients. These findings suggest the efficacy of orally administered antimeasles colostrum in improving the condition of MS patients. (Ebina)

Hyper-immune colostrum contains higher levels of antibodies than regular colostrum. I could not locate any studies using regular colostrum for MS so

I can not compare the benefits. It is possible that regular colostrum may not be as effective as hyper-immune colostrum in this case; however, some studies have shown that regular colostrum is just as effective as hyper-immune for certain conditions. (Clark)

IL-6 Levels and MS

Although IL-6 exhibits several proinflammatory activities, indirect evidence suggests that the cytokine may also play an immunomodulatory role in inflammatory demyelinating disorders such as MS. (Maimone)

One study at the Department of Neurology, at the Mayo Clinic in Rochester, Minnesota, showed that recombinant human IL-6 suppresses demyelination in a viral model of MS. Administration of human IL-6 (2.5 mcg, twice daily for 28 days) dramatically reduced demyelination and inflammation in the spinal cord of mice. Benefit also was observed when IL-6 was used as a therapeutic agent and begun on day 15 after infection, a time in which there is the first evidence of inflammation and demyelination in the spinal cord. Suppression of myelin damage by treatment with IL-6 was associated with fewer virus Ag-positive cells in the spinal cord. Infectious CNS virus levels were reduced in IL-6-treated animals on day 15 after infection, but not on day 7, 22 or 29 after infection. This suggests that this IL-6 may have an application for the treatment of human MS. (Rodriguez)

As lactoferrin provides regulatory effects on proinflammatory cytokines such as IL-6, it is possible that it may be of benefit.

Rheumatoid Arthritis

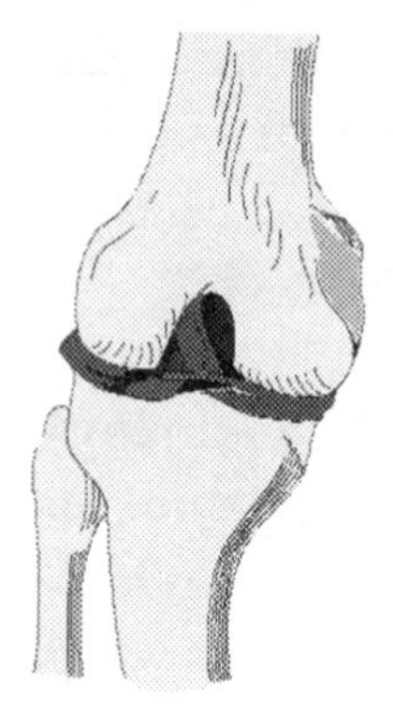

Rheumatoid arthritis is an autoimmune disease which causes chronic inflammation of the joints, the tissue around the joints, as well as other organs in the body. Autoimmune diseases are illnesses that occur when the body tissues are mistakenly attacked by its own immune system. The immune system is a complex organization of cells and antibodies designed normally to "seek and destroy" invaders of the body, particularly infections. Patients with these diseases have antibodies in their blood which target their own body tissues, where they can be associated with inflammation. Because it can affect multiple other organs of the body, rheumatoid arthritis is referred to as a systemic illness and is sometimes called rheumatoid disease. While rheumatoid arthritis is a chronic illness, meaning it can last for years, patients may experience long periods without symptoms.

Patients with rheumatoid arthritis have a defective suppressor T-cell system, and continue to make antibodies to a common virus, whereas the response normally shuts down after about a dozen days.

Rheumatoid arthritis is a common rheumatic disease, affecting more than two million people in the United States. The disease is three times more common in women as in men. It afflicts people of all races equally.

The cause of rheumatoid arthritis is largely unknown and there is no known cure.

Elevated levels of IL-6 in synovial fluid appears to reflect the local proinflammatory, potentially erosive activity in rheumatoid arthritis. (Van Leeuwen. Brennan, Punzi)

Lactoferrin Reduces Inflammatory Cytokines

Numerous studies, many conducted at the Institute of Immunology and Experimental Therapy, Polish Academy of Sciences, Weigla, Wroclaw, Poland, have been done to investigate the beneficial anti-inflammatory properties of orally ingested bovine lactoferrin.

In one study, rats with induced inflammation were given 5 oral doses of bovine lactoferrin (10 mg. each). The results revealed an inhibition of the induced inflammation in the bovine lactoferrin-treated rats by 50%. The inhibition was also associated with a substantial decrease in the ability of splenocytes to produce IL-6 in the bovine lactoferrin-treated rats (94%). TNF-alpha production was also decreased, although to a lesser degree (48%).

The researchers believed the decreased ability of spleen cells to produce inflammatory cytokines in bovine lactoferrin-treated rats may be the basis for the reduction in inflammation. (Zimecki)

Very low physiologic serum levels of lactoferrin increase significantly upon infection. Serum concentration of lactoferrin is also elevated in rheumatoid patients. Lactoferrin also diminishes the damaging effects of free radical release. Lactoferrin also controls the effector phase of cellular immune response and inhibits manifestations of autoimmune response in mice. (Adamik)

Fibromyalgia

While fibromyalgia is not yet officially classed as an auto-immune disorder, studies strongly suggest that it involves immune disregulation.

Fibromyalgia (also known as fibrositis) is a chronic condition causing pain, stiffness, and tenderness of the muscles, tendons, and joints. Fibromyalgia is also characterized by restless sleep, awakening feeling tired, fatigue, anxiety, depression and disturbances in bowel function.

While fibromyalgia is one of the most common diseases affecting the muscles, its cause is currently unknown. The painful tissues involved are not accompanied by tissue inflammation, tissue damage or deformity. Fibromyalgia also does not cause damage to internal body organs. This is unlike many other rheumatologic conditions (such as rheumatoid arthritis, systemic lupus and polymyositis).

Fibromyalgia affects predominantly women (90%) between the ages of 35 and 55. Although rarely, fibromyalgia can also affect men, children and the elderly. It can occur independently, or can occur with other conditions, such as lupus or arthritis.

The universal symptom of fibromyalgia is non-inflammatory-related pain. There seems to be an increased sensitivity to sensory stimuli, and an unusually low pain threshold. Minor sensory stimuli that ordinarily would not cause pain in individuals can cause disabling pain in individuals with fibromyalgia. Body pain can be aggravated by noise, weather change and emotional stress.

Fatigue occurs in 90% of individuals with

I am taking 6 colostrum-lactoferrin lozenges plus 3-6 glucosamine and MSM capsules daily. This, and a lot of prayer, has results in a significant decrease in the severity of my pain. I also am sleeping much better than I nomrally do in a flare-up. I don't know which one is helping, it might be all 3, but I am going to continue with all 3!
M.B.

fibromyalgia. Individuals also lack the deep, restorative level of sleep, called "non-rapid-eye-movement" (non-REM) sleep. Consequently, those with fibromyalgia often awaken in the morning without feeling fully rested.

Other common symptoms include poor concentration, forgetfulness, mood changes, irritability, migraine and tension headaches, numbness or tingling of different parts of the body, abdominal pain related to irritable bowel syndrome, and irritable bladder, causing painful and frequent urination. Like fibromyalgia, irritable bowel can cause chronic abdominal pain and other bowel disturbances without detectable inflammation of the stomach or the intestines. Fibromyalgia is often misdiagnosed as a psychological disorder.

Fibromyalgia and Immune Dysfunction

A number of researchers have shown that fibromyalgia has clear signs of immune dysfunction.

The results of a study conducted at the Department of Internal Medicine B, Carmel Medical Center, Haifa, Israel, suggest that there is a defect in the IL-2 pathway, which is related to protein kinase

C activation in patients with fibromyalgia. (Hader)

Researchers in Spain at the Hospital University Virgen Del Rocio, showed that the number of T-cells expressing activation markers CD69 and CD25 is decreased in patients with fibromyalgia. The results suggest a defect in T cell activation. (Hernanz)

Researchers in Poland found that individuals with fibromyalgia have similarities in leukocyte activity to individuals with allergies. They reported that allergy symptoms were found in about 50% of individuals with fibromyalgia. (Samborski)

Studies on sleep disorders and the symptoms of fibromyalgia showed a link between IL-1, immune-neuroendocrine-thermal systems and the sleep-wake cycle which results in nonrestorative sleep, pain, fatigue, cognitive and mood symptoms in patients with fibromyalgia. (Moldofsky)

These studies all suggest fibromyalgia involves immune disregulation. Therefore, colostrum and it's regulatory factors such as lactoferrin could be of great benefits. Hopefully, there will be clinical trials conducted in the near future so this can be demonstrated.

Part of having fibromyalgia is that I seemed to get every cold and flu that came around. After I started taking the colostrum and lactoferrin lozenges I noticed that I didn't get sick as often and that I had more energy. When I did get sick, it didn't seem like I was sick as long as I normaly would be or as long as other people were. The lozenges also may be helping my irritable bowel problems that I have been struggling with for years. (T.M.)

ULCERS, INFLAMMATORY BOWEL DISEASE & DIGESTIVE PROBLEMS

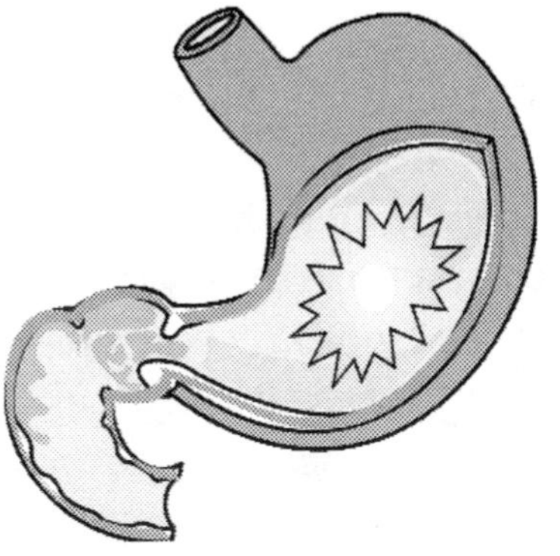

Peptic Ulcer

A peptic ulcer, also referred to as a gastric ulcer, is a sore or hole in the lining of the stomach or duodenum (the first part of the small intestine). People of any age can get an ulcer and women are affected just as often as men. Over 25 million Americans will suffer from an ulcer at some point during their lifetime.

Most ulcers are caused by the bacteria Helicobacter pylori (H. pylori); 90% of duodenal ulcers and more than 80% of gastric ulcers. Before 1982, when H. pylori was discovered, spicy food, acid, stress and lifestyle were considered the major causes of ulcers. The majority of patients were given long-term maintenance doses of acid-reducing medications, such as H2 blockers, without a chance for permanent cure.

H. pylori is found in the stomach of asymptomatic humans as well as patients with acid peptic disease and gastric adenocarcinoma. Many people who are infected with H. pylori do not suffer any symptoms related to the infection; however, it can cause chronic active, chronic persistent and atrophic gastritis in adults and children. Infected persons have a 2 to 6-fold increased risk of developing gastric cancer and mucosal-associated-lymphoid-type lymphoma compared with their uninfected counterparts - regardless of whether there are symptoms or not.

The most common ulcer symptom is gnawing or burning pain in the epigastrium. This pain typically occurs when the stomach is empty, between meals and in the early morning hours, but can also occur at other times. It may last from minutes to hours and may be relieved by eating or by taking antacids. Less common ulcer symptoms include nausea, vomiting, loss of appetite and bleeding. Prolonged bleeding may cause anemia leading to weakness and fatigue.

Bovine Colostrum Effective Against H. Pylori

Researchers at the Department of Clinical Pathology, Hospital for Sick Children, University of Toronto, Ontario, Canada, showed the benefits of bovine colostrum for ulcers caused by H. pylori.

They showed that bovine colostrum can block the binding of Helicobacter species to select lipids and that binding inhibition is conferred. Colostral lipids may interfere with adhesion of H. pylori to the lining of the stomach and intestinal tract therefore inhibit infection. (Bitzan)

Breast Feeding Inhibits H. Pylori Infection and Other Gastric Problems

Swedish researchers have demonstrated the importance of breast-feeding and its role in the protection against H. pylori infection in early life. (Stromqvist)

Researchers at the Department of Pediatrics, Ludwig-Maximilians University of Munich, Germany report that human milk provides a number of components (such as lactoferrin, growth factors, peptide and nonpeptide hormones, gastrointestinal regulatory peptides, etc.) are involved in the maturation of the gastrointestinal tract of the infant. In addition to the passive benefits provided by human milk, several data support the hypothesis that breast-feeding promotes the development of the infant's own immune system, which might confer long-term benefits for the newborn infant. The risk of IDDM (insulin-dependent diabetes), Crohn's disease, and atopic disease is lower in individuals who had been breast-fed during infancy. (Rodriguez-Palmero)

Other studies have also shown that human colostrum, and specifically secretory IgA, inhibits H. pylori adhesion. (Falk)

Researchers at Georgetown University Medical Center, Washington, D.C., in their discussion on infant protection against infectious diseases from

The risk of IDDM, Crohn's disease, and atopic disease is lower in individuals who had been breast-fed during infancy.

breast-feeding also describe the inhibition of H. pylori adhesion to the gastric mucosa by kappa-casein. (Hamosh)

Bovine Lactoferrin Effective Against H. Pylori

Researchers at the Department of Infectious Diseases, Tokai University School of Medicine, Kanagawa, Japan, showed bovine lactoferrin has a direct anti-bacterial effect on mice infected with H. pylori.

Mice orally inoculated with H. pylori were given 10 mg. bovine lactoferrin orally once daily. After 3 to 4 weeks the number of H. pylori in the stomach decreased to one-tenth. The lactoferrin also significantly inhibited the attachment of H. pylori to the stomach. As a result, the serum antibodies to H. pylori decreased to an undetectable level. The findings suggest that bovine lactoferrin exerts an inhibitory effect on colonizing H. pylori by detaching the bacterium from the gastric epithelium and by exerting a direct anti-bacterial effect. (Wada)

Researchers at the University of Texas-Houston Medical School also found antibiotic properties of bovine lactoferrin against H. pylori and stated that lactoferrin should be further investigated for possible use in human H. pylori infections and peptic ulcers. (Dial)

Human Studies on Lactoferrin and H. Pylori-Related Gastritis

Lactoferrin is present in gastric juice and levels somehow correlate with H. pylori infection. In a study made up of 30 individuals who were H. pylori-positive and 14 negative patients with chronic gastritis, they found that lactoferrin concentration in gastric juice was significantly higher in H. pylori-positive than in negative patients. Levels were higher even after correcting the lactoferrin levels for pH values or after adjusting the pH values of the gastric juice in both groups of patients as pH values are known to influence the levels of lactoferrin. In addition, the gastric juice levels of lactoferrin correlated significantly with the gastric mucosal concentrations of lactoferrin in the gastric body and the antrum. (Nakao)

These Japanese researchers also investigated the relationship between the gastric mucosal concentration of lactoferrin and H. pylori infection of the stomach. Their study was composed of 27 H. pylori-positive and 12 H. pylori-negative patients with chronic gastritis. The investigation showed, in vivo, that lactoferrin concentration is increased in patients with H. pylori-related gastritis, and that the levels of lactoferrin correlate significantly with the degree of inflammation of the gastric mucosa. The gastric mucosal level of lactoferrin may constitute an excellent marker of H. pylori infection. (Nakao)

Inflammatory Bowel Disease

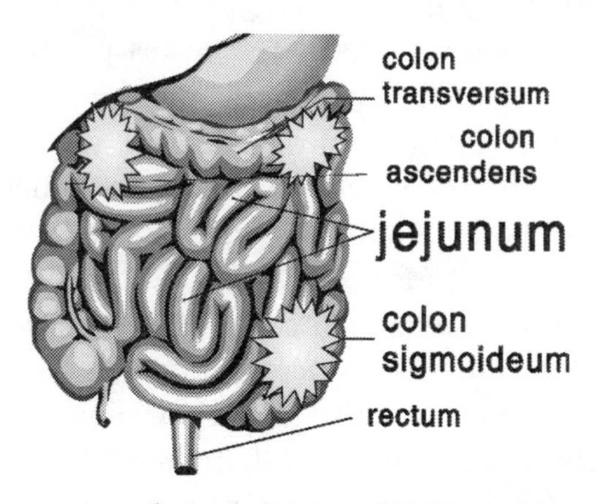

Inflammatory bowel disease (IBD) is a term used to describe two related diseases that involve inflammation of the small intestine (jejunum) and large intestine (colon): Ulcerative colitis and Crohn's disease. These are chronic inflammatory conditions that can last years to decades. IBD affects approximately 500,000 to 2 million people in the United States. Men and women are equally affected. IBD most commonly begins during adolescence and early adulthood, but it can also begin during childhood and later in life.

Ulcerative Colitis

Ulcerative colitis is a disease of the large intestine (colon). The colon is the part of the digestive system where waste material is stored. Individuals with ulcerative colitis, ulcers and inflammation of the inner lining of the colon lead to symptoms of abdominal pain, diarrhea and rectal bleeding. Ulcerative colitis is usually a chronic condition with symptoms lasting for months to years. It is most common in young adults, but can occur at any age. It is found worldwide, but is most common in the United States, England and northern Europe.

The exact cause of ulcerative colitis is unknown. Infection and allergy have been proposed as possible causes, but are not supported by research studies. Ulcerative colitis is currently believed to be an autoimmune disease, where the body tissues are attacked by its own immune system. In ulcerative colitis, the body's immune system is called upon to attack the inner lining of the large intestine, causing inflammation and ulceration.

The symptoms of ulcerative colitis vary according to the severity and extent of the disease. Some patients only have disease in the rectum (proctitis). Others have disease limited to the rectum and the adjacent left colon (proctosigmoiditis). Yet in others the entire colon is affected (universal colitis). Symptoms are generally more severe when a larger portion of the colon is involved. Individuals with universal colitis often have abdominal pain, diarrhea, rectal bleeding, weight loss, fever, loss of appetite and other more serious complications.

Enteroinvasive E. coli (EIEC) is a class of infectious bacteria that can adhere to and invade the intestinal wall, kill intestinal cells and produce inflammation in the colon, generally referred to as colitis. The most renowned strain, E. coli 0157:H7, causes bloody diarrhea, also known as hemorrhagic colitis. There is no treatment for E. coli infection.

Components in colostrum are known to effectively block the damaging effects of E. coli 0157:H7 in humans. The high levels of colostrum antibodies and neutralizing activity against important disease-causing factors of E. coli O157 make colostrum an excellent potential therapeutic in the treatment of diarrhea and the prevention of E. coli-associated complications. (Lissner)

Crohn's Disease

Crohn's disease involves chronic inflammation of the intestines. Common symptoms of Crohn's disease include abdominal pain, diarrhea and weight loss. Less common symptoms include poor appetite, fever, night sweats, rectal pain and rectal bleeding. Like ulcerative colitis, the symptoms and the prognosis of Crohn's disease are dependent on the location and the intensity of the inflammation.

While ulcerative colitis appears only in the colon and the rectum, Crohn's disease affects the colon, the rectum and the small intestine. In rare instances, Crohn's disease can also involve the stomach, the mouth and the esophagus (located between the mouth and the stomach). Like ulcerative colitis, there are different types of Crohn's disease based on disease locations.

Except in the most severe cases, the inflammation in ulcerative colitis tends to involve the superficial layers of the inner wall. The inflammation tends also to be diffuse and uniform (all the mucosa in the affected segment of the bowel is inflamed). Unlike ulcerative colitis, the Crohn's disease inflammation is more localized and involves deeper layers of the intestinal wall.

Elevated Proinflammatory Cytokines Seen in Inflammatory Bowel Diseases

Cytokine secretion, which is important in the regulation of normal gastrointestinal immune responses, appears to be dysregulated in inflammatory bowel diseases. Numerous studies show that individuals with either Crohn's disease or ulcerative colitis display high levels of NF-kappa B DNA-binding activity accompanied by an increased production of IL-1, IL-6, and TNF-alpha. (Neurath, McClane, Rogler, Ishiguro) These proinflammatory cytokines are believed to be involved in the cause of ulcerative colitis. (Ishiguro)

I am 61. About 10 years ago I was treated for rectal cancer. Though the treatment was successful, it left me with radiation proctitus, which causes regular soreness, irritation and elimination difficulties. From the first day I starting taking colostrum and lactoferrin lozenges, I have experienced significant healing of the radiation proctitus.

Also, the colostrum/lactoferrin seems to have straightened out many other digeative problems that I have had for years. I have been able to discontinue taking hydrochloric acid tablets, which I had to take to compensate for a lack of stomach acid. I can even eat Mexican food at night and get a good night's sleep instead of lying awake with stomach distress.

I also have a chronic respiratory illness. I am convinced by the increased feeling of well-being that the product is helping my immune system.

Thank you, N.S.

As studies have shown that lactoferrin is helpful in the regulation of immune responses, and specifically the down production of proinflammatory cytokines, IL-1, IL-6 and TNF-alpha (Zimecki), it is possible that lactoferrin supplementation could be highly beneficial. I have not found any published clinical trials with lactoferrin supplementation and these conditions. Hopefully, there will be in the near future.

Irritable Bowel Syndrome

Irritable bowel syndrome (IBS) also called "spastic colon," is one of the most common gastrointestinal disorders. It has also been called spastic colitis, mucus colitis or nervous colon syndrome. It is characterized by abdominal pain, bloating, mucous in stools and irregular bowel habits, including alternating diarrhea and constipation. It tends to be a chronic disorder. Some individuals experience alternating episodes of relapse and improvement.

Up to 15% of the population may have IBS, affecting women about twice as often as men. The symptoms of IBS typically occur early in life, and half of the patients have onset of symptoms before they reach 30 years of age.

IBS is thought to be the result of abnormal contractions of the large intestine (colon). The cause(s) of such altered intestinal motility is not known. Dietary, psychological, hormonal or genetic factors may each play a role. In some patients, excessive contractions lead to spasms in the colon, causing abdominal pain, diarrhea or constipation. Other patients with irritable bowel syndrome are believed to have increased nervous sensitivity to normal events that occur in the intestine during digestion.

Symptoms of IBS usually begin during adolescence or early adulthood. Altered bowel movements occur over periods of days to weeks. Occasionally, symptoms may be continuous.

During episodes of constipation, stools may be hard, small, pebble-like and difficult to eliminate. This may be associated with a sense of incomplete evacuation. Passage of stool or gas may lead to the alleviation of pain.

The diarrhea of IBS is usually of small volume, but frequent. Episodes commonly occur during periods of stress. There is usually no associated fever or rectal bleeding.

From my clinical experience I have found that many "irritable bowel" patients suffer from small amounts of "gut seepage". This seepage manifests in "leaky gut syndrome". In extreme cases, people suffer from clinical disorders that cause ulcerations–some due to actions by microorganisms.

I have found that the IGF-1 and other factors in colostrum have helped "seal" the gut from ulceration in a number of patients. Included in an immuno-enhancement protocol, colostrum may be the key to pathogen removal and intestinal healing.

Kenneth D. Johnson, S.M.D., S.N.D., O.M.D., Ph.D., International Orthomolecular Nutritionist

Abdominal pain can vary in severity from mild to severe. It is usually felt in the lower abdomen, especially on the left side. The pain may be dull or sharp; crampy or continuous.

Other symptoms include abdominal distention, belching or a sensation of bloating. On rare occasions, heartburn, nausea and vomiting are seen.

Depression, anxiety and stress are commonly associated with IBS. Stress can cause a reactivation of previous enteric inflammation. Stress can also enhance the response to subsequent inflammatory stimuli (Collins) and is often believed to be a trigger of returning difficulty during periods of improvement.

Inflammation of the intestine causes pain and altered motility. Inflammation of the mucosa of the gastrointestinal tract is accompanied by changes in enteric nerve and smooth muscle function, and in gut motility and sensation.

The causes of IBS are largely unknown. One prevailing theory is that partially undigested proteins irritate the upper intestinal tract, sometimes referred to as "leaky gut syndrome." Another possible cause is suspected to be irritation caused by bacterial or parasite infection.

Dr. Kenneth Johnson of San Jose, California, reports that he has had success with a number of patients with irritable bowel using colostrum and lactoferrin involving either cause. Studies do suggest that anti-inflammatory therapy may be beneficial for individuals with IBS (Sanovic, Collins) opening the door of possibility for lactoferrin treatment.

I have heard of number of personal testimonies from individuals with IBS supplementing colostrum lactoferrin lozenges who experienced improvement of symptoms, but could find no published clinical studies in this area.

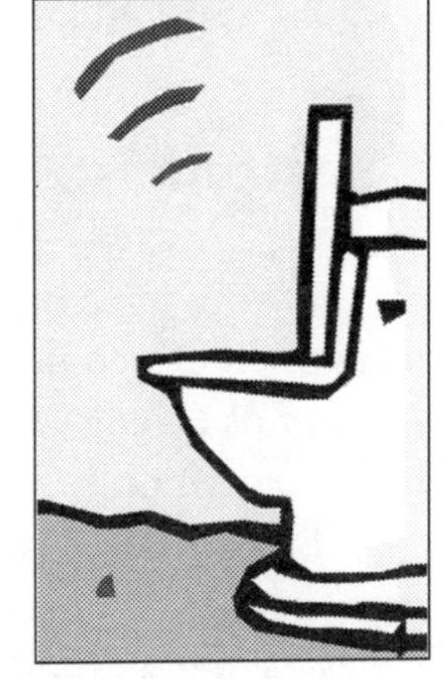

Diarrhea

Diarrhea refers to unusually frequent or liquid bowel movements. Diarrhea is the opposite of constipation. There are many causes of diarrhea, which can be divided into two major categories – infectious and noninfectious. Infectious causes of diarrhea are a result of abnormal microorganisms (bacteria, viruses or parasites) invading the bowels.

Bacteria capable of causing diarrhea:

- Clostridrium difficile (bacteria found in feces of newborns)
- Escherichia coli (E. coli - from contaminated food, water and infected food handlers)
- Salmonella (the agents of typhoid fever and many other diseases)
- Gastroenteritis and enteric fever (from contaminated food products)
- Shigella (a cause of epidemic bacillary dysentery)
- Campylobacter (another food-handler's contaminant)

- Vibrio cholerae (the agent of cholera - an acute bacterial infections of the intestinal tract. The mortality rate is 50% if untreated. The bacteria is spread by contaminated people or food)

Colostrum is Effective Against E. Coli

E. coli is a bacteria that normally lives in the intestines of people and animals and elsewhere. Most strains of E. coli are quite harmless. E. coli 0157:H7 is an exception.

E. coli 0157:H7 is a major health problem as a dangerous, disease-causing bacteria. About 20,000 cases of hemorrhagic colitis (bloody diarrhea) due to E. coli 0157:H7 occur each year in the United States. E. coli 0157:H7 comes mostly from unsanitary cooking conditions, poorly cooked food (particularly hamburger) and contaminated water from untreated wells, streams or lakes.

E. coli 0157:H7 struck at least 8 youngsters who played in a wading pool in Atlanta in 1998. It caused kidney failure in four of the children.

E. coli 0157:H7 causes bloody diarrhea (hemorrhagic colitis), hemolytic-uremic syndrome (a blood and kidney disease in children), and thrombotic thrombocytic purpura (a dire disease in the elderly). There is no specific treatment for E. coli infection.

In 1996, German researchers showed that components in colostrum from non-immunized cows were able to effectively block the damaging effects of E. coli in humans. They stated that since colostrum contains high levels of antibodies and neutralizing activity against important disease-causing factors of E. coli.

This has potential use in the treatment of diarrhea and the prevention of E. coli-associated complications. (Lissner)

In a placebo-controlled, double-blind study with individuals with E. coli-associated diarrhea, stool frequencies in the group treated with bovine colostrum were significantly reduced compared with those in the placebo group. No side effects were attributable to the colostrum treatment. (Huppertz)

Colostrum and lactoferrin are also effective against a number of other bacteria that are known to cause diarrhea.

Colostrum Effective Against Diarrhea-producing Viruses

Many viruses common in our everyday lives, can cause diarrhea. During their first 5 years of life, almost all children acquire rotavirus (which causes inflammation of the stomach and bowels causing intestinal disease).

In the double-blind, placebo-controlled trial, 80 children with rotavirus diarrhea orally received either 10 g. of bovine colostrum daily for 4 days or a placebo. Children who received bovine colostrum had significantly less daily and total stool output and stool frequency and required a smaller amount of oral rehydration solution than did children who received the placebo. Clearance of rotavirus from the stool was also earlier in the colostrum group compared with the placebo group (average days, 1.5 vs. 2.9). No adverse reactions from the colostrum treatment were observed. (Sarker)

Colostrum Effective Against Diarrhea-producing Parasites

Colostrum has shown to be highly effective against many of the major parasites including:

- Cryptosporidium parvum (a major cause of diarrhea in immunodeficient persons)

- Entamoeba histolytica (which causes ameobic dysentery)

- Giardia lamblia (which causes malabsorption of fluids in the bowels and speeds contents through the intestines to produce diarrhea. By age 5, many children have acquired Giardia.)

Food poisoning, irritable bowel syndrome, and Crohn's disease are among other noninfectious causes of diarrhea.

Diarrhea was discussed earlier in the section on HIV/AIDS, but obviously everyone who gets diarrhea does not have HIV. HIV simply makes one at a higher risk for infection of a diarrhea-causing microorganism.

Studies done on individuals with diarrhea who were otherwise healthy also show that supplemental bovine colostrum is very effective.

CHOLESTEROL & HEART DISEASE

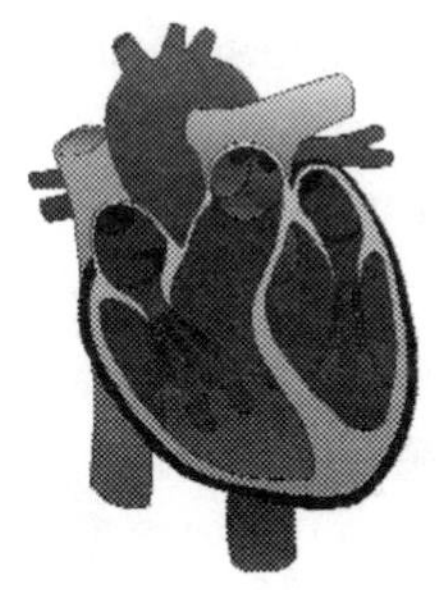

Cholesterol is a fatty chemical that is an important part of the outer lining (membrane) of cells in the body. Most cholesterol is produced in the liver, and is carried in the bloodstream to the body's cells by special proteins called "lipoproteins." Cholesterol has the properties of an oil and cannot dissolve in blood without lipoproteins. The two major lipoproteins are low density lipoprotein (LDL) and high density lipoprotein (HDL). Dietary cholesterol is found mainly in animal-based foods such as beef, poultry (especially liver) and dairy products.

LDL cholesterol is called the "bad" cholesterol because elevated LDL levels are associated with an

> *Colostrum proline-rich polypeptide may have a role in reversing heart disease very much like it does with allergies and autoimmune diseases. Altered immunity may be the hidden cause of atherosclerosis and cardiovascular disease. A "New England Journal of Medicine" article indicated that heart disease is partially the result of immune sensitization to cardiac antigens. Therefore, I generally include colostrum in all immune-enhancement and cardiac programs.*
>
> *Kenneth D. Johnson, S.M.D., S.N.D., O.M.D., Ph.D., International Orthomolecular Nutritionist*

increased risk of coronary heart disease. LDL deposits cholesterol on the artery walls, causing the formation of a hard, thick substance called cholesterol plaque. Over time, this plaque causes thickening of the artery walls and narrowing of the arteries, called atherosclerosis.

Coronary arteries narrowed by plaque are incapable of supplying enough blood and oxygen to the heart muscle during exertion. Lack of oxygen (ischemia) to the heart muscle causes chest pain. A blood clot in the artery can cause complete blockage of the artery, leading to death of heart muscle (heart attack).

Coronary artery disease is the most common cause of death in the United States, accounting for about 600,000 deaths annually.

Lactoferrin Inhibits Cholesterol Accumulation

Plaque buildup involves free radical damage associated with oxidized LDL cholesterol caused by macrophage accumulation. Japanese researchers showed that lactoferrin inhibits the accumulation of oxidized cholesterol in a dose-dependent manner. In the presence of bovine lactoferrin, oxidized cholesterol accumulation decreased by more than 80%.

Interestingly, the study showed that human lactoferrin was less potent than bovine lactoferrin. The results indicated that lactoferrin inhibits the binding of modified LDLs to macrophages by direct interaction with modified LDLs, resulting in their loss of function as ligands of the scavenger receptor. The results suggest that lactoferrin in the blood stream may act as an anti-atherogenic agent. (Kajikawa)

DENTAL HEALTH

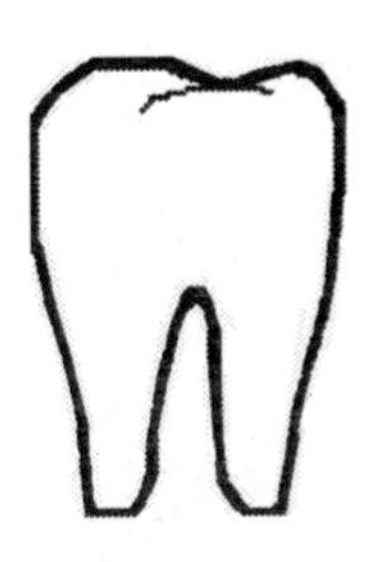

Cavities

Cavities (also known as caries or tooth decay) is the progressive deterioration of teeth or bones. Caries is usually accompanied by inflammation of the surrounding soft tissue. Bacteria are always present in the mouth. But when food becomes trapped between the teeth, the bacteria break it down and form a harmful acid capable of softening the enamel and eroding the teeth.

Saliva Has Natural Antibacterial Effects on Cavity-Causing Bacteria

Our saliva was carefully designed to protect our teeth and gums. It contains many antimicrobial agents (including lactoferrin) which are known to have anti-bacterial effects on cavity-causing bacteria, in particular against Streptococcus mutans.

Studies by researchers in Finland have shown that enhancing these properties of saliva can be done by adding antimicrobial proteins such as peroxidase, lactoferrin and lysozyme to oral health products. The researchers stated that although clinical evidence is still limited, the idea of using such "natural antibiotics" rather than synthetic agents against cavity-causing bacteria seems promising. (Tenovuo)

Colostrum and lactoferrin in a liquid or lozenge would be protective in the same way.

Periodontal Disease

Periodontal disease, sometimes called gingivitis or gum disease, involves inflammation and degradation of the soft tissue (gingiva) and abnormal loss of bone that surrounds the teeth and holds them in place. Gum disease is caused by toxins secreted by bacteria in "plaque" that accumulate over time along the gum line. This plaque is a mixture of food, saliva and bacteria. If this remains on the teeth, calcium salts begin to form and build up a hard, chalky deposit around the teeth known as tartar. Although careful cleaning and flossing can remove the particles of food that encourage plaque, no amount of cleaning can remove tartar. Once it is there, the dentist or hygienist has to scale the teeth to get rid of it.

Early symptoms include gum bleeding without pain. Pain is a symptom of more advanced gum disease as the loss of bone around the teeth leads to the formation of gum pockets. Bacteria in these pockets cause gum infection, swelling, pain and further bone destruction. Advanced gum disease can cause loss of otherwise healthy teeth.

I have been taking the colostrum and lactoferrin lozenges for some time. Then I realized one day that my gums were no longer bleeding when I was brushing my teeth. This has been a problem I was having for quite a while, which is one of the early signs of periodontal disease. I will keep taking them for that reason alone!

Thank you, K.M

Lactoferrin May Benefit Dry Mouth

As we get older, the production of saliva and the protective lactoferrin it contains decreases. This is one of the reasons that periodontal disease is so common.

Individuals with various autoimmune conditions are also at a higher risk for development of dental problem. Sjogren's syndrome, also known as dry mouth or xerostomia, often accompanies conditions such as arthritis, diabetes, lupus, etc. As the body defense system is upset with the autoimmune disorder, it begins to destroy the glands that produce lubricating secretions.

Dry mouth can also be caused by aging, smoking, pregnancy, stress and medical conditions such as hypertension and cancer. Dry mouth can also result from chemotherapy and radiation treatment to the throat or mouth areas or may result as a side effect of many common medications. These include:

Analgesics (pain relievers)

Anti-histimines (often taken for colds, hayfever and allergies)

Anti-cholinergics (i.e., hyoscyamine, which reduces spasms of the digestive system, bladder and urethra)

Anti-arrhythmics (taken for irregular heart beat, i.e., amiodarone or Cordarone®)

Anti-hypertensives (taken for high blood pressure, i.e., Minipress® or Aldomet® or methyldopa)

Anti-depressants (taken for depression or sleep problems, i.e., amitripytline or Elavil®, Xanax®, Desyrel®, Asendin®, etc.)

Diuretics (taken to reduce water retention, i.e., Dyazide®, Aldactone® and Enduron®)

Tranquilizers (used for anxiety and stress, i.e., Ataraz®, Centrax®, Mellaril® and Tranxene®)

Whenever the flow of protective saliva is inhibited, the risk of dental problems increases. Periodontal disease and cavies are prevalent among individuals with dry mouth. Dry mouth can also cause problems in speaking, swallowing and eating.

Lactoferrin in a liquid, lozenge or spray, or added to mouth rinse, tooth paste or other dental type product may be helpful to prevent problems associated with dry mouth.

Lactoferrin Inhibits Periodontal Bacteria

Researchers have shown that both human and bovine lactoferrin inhibited the adhesion of periodontitis-associated bacteria. The inhibitory effect was dose-dependent. In the presence of lactoferrin, decreased association of bacteria with the cell monolayers was also found. The researchers stated that their findings indicate that lactoferrin may prevent the establishment of bacteria in periodontal tissues through adhesion-counteracting mechanisms in addition to its anti-bacterial properties. (Alugupalli)

Researchers at the University of Lund, Sweden, also demonstrated the binding effects of human lactoferrin on various bacterial strains associated with periodontal disease, P. intermedia strains, P. gingivalis and P. melaninogenica. (Kalfas)

Place a drop or two of colostrum-lactoferrin liquid directly on the affected area. If liquid is not available, the contents of colostrum-lactoferrin capsule can be emptied, placing the powder directly on inflamed infected gum tissue.

Lactoferrin Inhibits Candida Albicans (Thrush)

Candida albicans is a yeast-like fungus that inhabits the intestines, mouth, genital tract and throat. Normally this fungus lives in balance with the other bacteria and yeasts in the body. However, certain conditions can cause this fungus to multiply out of control, weakening the immune system and causing an infection known as candidiasis. This infection can occur any where in the body, most frequently in the mouth (called thrush), the vagina (called vaginitis), gastrointestinal tract, ears or nose. Jock itch, athletes foot and diaper rash may also be forms of Candida albicans infections. Intense itching usually accompanies most of these infections.

In the oral cavity, white sores may form on the tongue, gums and inside the cheeks. There may also be pain with swallowing.

The use of broad spectrum antibiotics and immunodeficieny are often associated with Candida infection.

A number of studies have demonstrated that bovine lactoferrin is able to inhibit the growth of Candida albicans. (Wakabayashi, Xu, Vorland) Japanese researchers showed that both human and bovine lactoferrin increased the action of neutrophils to inhibit Candida growth. (Wakabayash) The Chinese researchers demonstrated lactoferrin's inhibitory effect of Candida specifically in the oral cavity. (Xu)

It is possible that topical applications could be beneficial as well for athletes foot, diaper rash, vaginitis and other similar problems.

Potential Application for Oral Care Products

German researchers have pointed out that peptides derived from bovine and human lactoferrin, have antimicrobial activity against oral pathogens and also that both peptides from bovine lactoferrin had more potent antimicrobial activities (against both Gram-positive and Gram-negative bacteria) than the human equivalents. The researchers stated that bovine lactoferrin should be investigated for use in oral care products. (Groenink)

> *I am 75 years old and have been taking colostrum-lactoferrin lozenges for some time. It must be helping my immune system because I do not get the colds and flu viruses that everyone else around me seems to get. My whole family is taking the lozenges and none of them have been sick either.*
>
> *But I think even more remarkable is the colostrum-lactoferrin spray/liquid. I had been experiencing inflammation and pain on the whole right side of my jaw for several months. It was very painful to chew. I was concerned that I was developing an abscess. I used one or two sprays a day for just two days and it was completely healed. It was unbelievable. I can't wait to tell my dentist as all he could recommend was to use salt water, which did nothing. Everyone should know how wonderful colostrum-lactoferrin spray is!*
>
> *Thank you, I.G.*

DIABETES

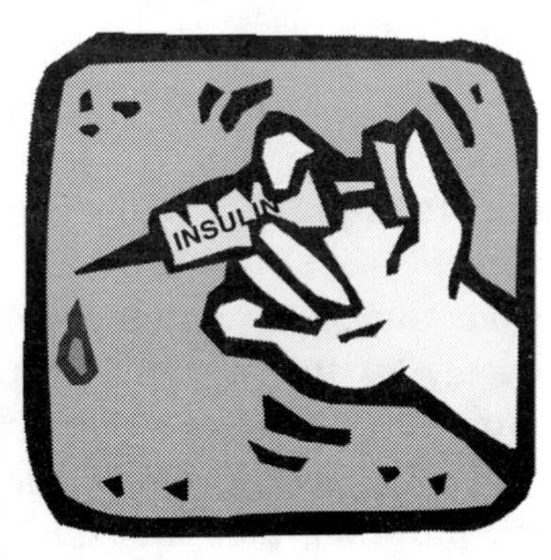

Diabetes mellitus is a chronic medical condition associated with abnormally high levels of sugar (glucose) in the blood. Elevated levels of blood glucose (hyperglycemia) lead to spillage of glucose into the urine, hence the term sweet urine. Normally, blood glucose levels are tightly controlled by insulin, a hormone produced by the pancreas. Insulin lowers the blood glucose level. When the blood glucose elevates (for example, after eating food), insulin is released from the pancreas to normalize the glucose level. In patients with diabetes mellitus, the absence or insufficient production of insulin causes hyperglycemia.

Diabetes mellitus is a chronic medical condition, meaning it can last a life time. Over time, diabetes mellitus can lead to blindness, kidney failure and nerve damage. Diabetes is also an important factor in accelerating the hardening and narrowing of the arteries (atherosclerosis), leading to strokes, coronary heart diseases and other blood vessel diseases in the body.

Diabetes affects 12 million people (6% of the population) in the United States. The direct and indirect cost of diabetes mellitus is $40 billion per year. It is the third leading cause of death in the United States after heart disease and cancer.

What Causes Diabetes?

The lack of insulin, insufficient production of insulin, production of defective insulin or the inability of cells to use insulin leads to hyperglycemia and diabetes mellitus. Glucose is a simple sugar found in food. Glucose is an essential nutrient that provides energy for the proper functioning of the body cells. After meals, food is digested in the stomach and the intestines. The glucose in digested food is absorbed by the intestinal cells into the bloodstream, and is carried by blood to all the cells in the body. However, glucose cannot enter the cells alone. It needs assistance from insulin to penetrate the cell walls. Without insulin, cells become starved of glucose energy despite the presence of abundant glucose in the blood. The abundant, unutilized glucose is wastefully excreted in the urine.

Juvenile diabetes (Type I, insulin dependent) is thought to result from an autoimmune mechanism, possibly initiated by an allergic reaction to the protein GAD found in cow's milk. Colostrum contains several factors that can offset this and other allergies. Colostrum IgF-1 can bind to both the insulin and IgF-1 receptors found on all cells. Human trials in 1990 reported that IgF-1 stimulates glucose utilization, effectively treating acute hyperglycemia and lessening a Type II diabetic's dependence on insulin. For these reasons I feel colostrum should be a part of every protocol for hyperglycemia and diabetes.

Kenneth D. Johnson, S.M.D., S.N.D., O.M.D., Ph.D., International Orthomolecular Nutritionist

Insulin is a hormone that is produced by specialized cells (islet cells) of the pancreas. In addition to helping glucose enter the cells, insulin is also important in tightly regulating the level of glucose in the blood. After a meal, the blood glucose level rises. In response to the increased glucose level, the pancreas normally releases insulin into the bloodstream to help glucose enter the cells and lower blood glucose levels. When the blood glucose levels are lowered, the insulin release from the pancreas is turned off. In normal individuals, such a regulatory system helps to keep blood glucose levels in a tightly controlled range.

In diabetics, the insulin is either missing (as in Type I diabetes mellitus), or insulin regulation is defective and insufficient (as in Type II diabetes mellitus). Both cause elevated levels of blood glucose (hyperglycemia).

Type I diabetes mellitus is also called insulin dependent diabetes mellitus (IDDM), or juvenile onset diabetes mellitus. In Type I diabetes mellitus, the pancreas releases no insulin at all, and the patient relies on insulin medication for survival.

Abnormal antibodies have been found in patients with IDDM. Antibodies are proteins in the blood that are part of the body's immune system. Normally, the immune system is designed to protect the body against foreign invaders and infections. In autoimmune diseases, such as IDDM, the immune system mistakenly manufactures antibodies that are directed against and cause damage to patients' own body tissues. It is believed that the tendency to develop these abnormal antibodies in IDDM is genetically inherited.

Type II diabetes mellitus is also referred to as

non-insulin dependent diabetes mellitus (NIDDM), or adult onset diabetes mellitus (AODM). In Type II diabetes, patients can still produce insulin, but do so inadequately. The pancreas in these patients not only produces an insufficient amount of insulin, but also releases insulin late in response to increased glucose levels. Some Type II diabetics have body cells that are resistant to the action of insulin. Finally, the liver in these patients continues to produce glucose despite elevated glucose levels. Type II diabetes occurs mostly in individuals over 40 years old.

The incidence of Type II diabetes increases with age. Unlike Type I diabetes mellitus, the majority of Type II diabetic patients are obese. Type II diabetes mellitus also has a strong genetic tendency.

Diabetes mellitus can also occur transiently during pregnancy. IGF-1 levels are lower in diabetic pregnant women compared to nondiabetic pregnant women. (DiBiase)

I am a diabetic in the advanced stages, I have an autoimmune disease, cardiovascular disease, have have multiple surgeries over the last 4 years and needless to say wasn't in very good health.

After taking colostrum and lactoferrin lozenges for about two months and my eyes actually started to improve after 4 years of degration.

My overall health has improved. Every year for as long I can remember I have horrible bronchial problems starting in October. It's now past January and I haven't had a problem yet!

Thank you, T.M.

IGF-1 and Insulin

Insulin-like growth factor-I (IGF-I) can stimulate glucose utilization in nondiabetic subjects and that the action of the IGF-I receptor is normal in the skeletal muscle of patients with NIDDM, it seems possible that IGF-I might provide an effective acute treatment for the hyperglycemia of NIDDM. Studies have shown that plasma levels of IGF-I in diabetic patients are lower than those in either of the nondiabetic groups. (Dohm)

Depressed levels of IGF-1 increases cellular and tissue sensitivity. Low IGF-1 levels are associated with many of the complications of diabetes, especially in Type II diabetes (Cortizo), such as kidney problems (Segev), weight gain and obesity (Bereket), diabetic retinopathy (Lacka), injury and delayed wound healing (Brown) and possibly vascular complications and cardiovascular disease (Goke, Bereket).

Researchers at the Department of Medicine, University of Miami School of Medicine, Florida, have shown that as IGF-1 decreases collagen degradation and therefore, IGF-1 may have beneficial implications for diabetic complications. (Lupia)

Researchers at the Department of Pediatrics, John Radcliffe Hospital, Oxford, UK, showed that addition of IGF-I treatment to insulin in adolescents with IDDM can restore circulating IGF-I levels and thus suppress GH levels and improve insulin sensitivity and glycemic control and decreases insulin requirements. (Dunger)

Can the IGF-1 in colostrum benefit diabetics?

Several studies show that bovine colostrum supplementation increases serum IGF-1. (Mero, Wester)

Dr. Raymond Lombardi reports that the diabetic patients in his Alternative Health Care Practice in Redding, California, who are taking 3-6 colostrum-lactoferrin lozenges daily all report fasting glucose reading an average of 10 points lower. They also report a reduced frequency in infection.

Other diabetic individuals using colostrum-lactoferrin lozenges report the following:

- Within 3 days, fasting blood sugar levels upon awakening are normal.
- Within 7 days, insulin use is reduced to 1/2.
- Within 30 days, their fingernails have hardened.

Lactoferrin May Improve Diabetics' Resistance to Infection and Tissue Damage

Diabetics have an increased susceptibility to bacterial infections. This is associated with abnormally high levels of advanced glycation end-products (AGEs) in tissue and serum that may inhibit antibacterial proteins such as lactoferrin and lysosyme.

Studies show that diabetics (as well as aging animals) have increased concentrations of AGEs in their collagen. AGEs are very damaging to collagen, which is found in the skin, blood vessels and connective tissue. This is responsible for accelerated tissue aging in proteins such as collagen and myelin in diabetics. It is believed to be responsible for complications of diabetes such as kidney damage and atherosclerosis.

Lactoferrin specifically binds to glucose-modified

proteins bearing AGEs. Exposure to AGE-modified proteins blocks the bacterial killing activities of lactoferrin and also inhibits the bactericidal and enzymatic activity of lysozyme. The researchers at the Picower Institute for Medical Research, Manhasset, New York, uncovering these results determined that this information may provide a basis for the development of new approaches to prevent diabetic infections. (Li)

It is possible that supplementation of lactoferrin may increase antibacterial activity and decrease one's risk of infection, while human studies need to be conducted to prove this.

Studies show that lactoferrin levels are similar in diabetics compared to non-diabetics, however, research shows that the effectiveness of lactoferrin to fight off bacteria in diabetics is significantly diminished. (Muratsu)

Periodontal Disease in Diabetics

A higher prevalence and severity of periodontal disease is detected in diabetic individuals. A number of studies have reported significantly lower resting salivary flow rates in IDDM compared to NIDDM or controls. (Ben-Aryeh)

Changes in the concentrations of total protein, albumin, lysozyme and lactoferrin in whole resting saliva have also been seen. (Ben-Aryeh)

As a Vietnam Veteran, I was exposed to Agent Orange. I had a high blood sugar count when I was discharged from the service. Six years later I became insulin dependent due to pancreatic failure. For the last 20 years I have lived as a brittle diabetic. I have experienced loss of sight in one eye and numerous other medical complications due to my illness.

I have been taking colostrum and lactoferrin lozenges for the last 2 months. since then I have noticed the following:

- *Dosage of insulin required reduced to 1/2*
- *Improved energy*
- *Increased alertness*
- *Better sleep patterns*
- *Lowered stress levels*
- *Elimination of colds and illness*
- *Promoted healing of cuts and bruises*
- *Stopped splitting of finger and toe nails.*

This has definitely had a phenomenal impact on my life.

Thank you, S.B.

BENEFITS FOR ATHLETES

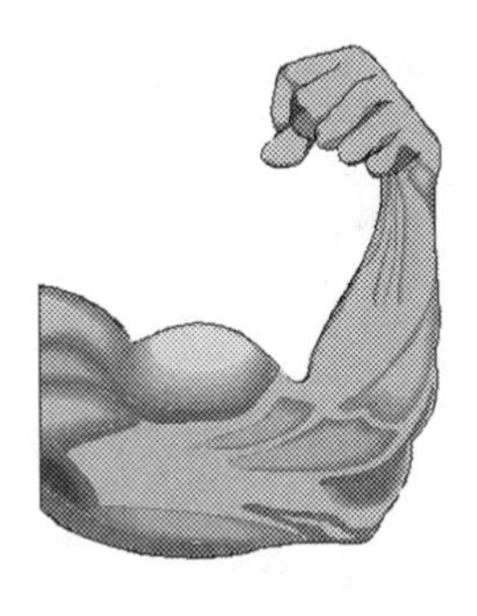

For years athletes have been interested in colostrum because of the Insulin-like Growth Factor I and II (IGF-I and IGF-II) it contains. These are pro-insulin hormones that have anabolic (muscle promoting) effects. They are composed of an amino acid chain that resembles the hormone insulin.

Both bovine and human colostrum growth factors have demonstrated the ability to stimulate protein synthesis and inhibit protein degradation. (Francis, Rinderkneckt, Humbel) IGF-1 in bovine colostrum contains the identical amino acid sequence except for a 26 amino acid segment on the front of the bovine molecule which, when split by digestive acids in our stomach, releases a highest concentrations of IGF-I available in nature.

The primary function of IGF-1 and II in colostrum is to promote rapid tissue growth through protein synthesis of the newborn. Makes sense, right?

In adults, IGF-1 and IGF-II are important factors involved in cell proliferation and metabolism, regulation of tissue repair, growth and differentiation. Remember that our tissues are in a constant state of repair. In the athlete, this is of critical significance, because the damage is also a result of hard training. This results in "soreness," which can interfere with performance and training, so quick healing is highly desirable. In the bodybuilder, muscle growth only occurs as the tissue is repairing itself.

IGF-1 is released by many different tissues throughout the body and affects almost every cell to some degree. Major organs that synthesize IGF-1 are the heart, lungs, kidneys, liver, pancreas, spleen, small intestines, testes, ovaries, large intestines, brain, bone, pituitary and human placenta.

The majority of IGF-1 is secreted by the liver in response to a signal from human growth hormone (hGH). The major target tissues affected by the IGF-1 in combination with the human growth hormone (HgH) signal are muscle, cartilage, bone, liver, kidney, nerves, skin and lungs.

IGF-1 assists cells toward cell division and the ability to complete DNA synthesis. IGF-1 not only helps cell growth by division, but also by enhancing cell specialization. IGF-1 communicates an anabolic signal to cells, regulating cell division and differentiation as the muscle acquires an increased need for strength or as injury to the muscle is incurred. IGF-1 promotes the growth of muscle and bone.

IGF-1 acts within the nervous system and is critical for the growth and development of nerve cells. IGF-1 maintains a high level of cell communication at the neuromuscular junction, where the cooperation between the nerve and muscle cells take place.

IGF-1 is believed to bring aging, resting cells back into a balanced state optimizing cell activity and tissue performance.

Hormonal functions such as the anabolic (constructive) activity of HgH depends on the production and presence of IGF-1 to achieve positive results. IGF-

I stimulates growth of tissues by increasing the number of cells: growth hormone increases their size. (Burke)

Other growth factors present in colostrum include epidermal growth factor, platelet-derived growth factor and transforming growth factor-beta. Each of these is capable of stimulating cell division and tissue development. (Burke)

The following are associated with IGF-1:

- Increased physical performance
- Increased mental performance
- Increased physical endurance
- Increase in lean muscle tissue growth
- Wound healing and repair

Colostrum Research Shos Benefits to Athletes

Many colostrum users report decreased recovery time and decreased soreness after acute exercise when using a colostrum supplement. This is, of course subjective, but there is some scientific evidence that support these claims.

Anabolic and tissue repair functions of insulin-like growth factors have been studied extensively, and it seems that healing of injuries and post-workout recovery are improved as well with IGF-1 supplementation.

Obviously the anti-inflammatory benefits of colostrum/lactoferrin are of great interest to the athlete, but increased nutrient absorption is also of significance. IGF-1 is also important for its affect on development, diabetes and other chronic diseases.

Some colostrum manufacturer advertisements have featured scientific research reports showing that the high levels of growth factors in colostrum clearly enhance cell growth in the test tube, which, by inference, suggests that colostrum will enhance muscle growth and thus athletic performance.

Faster Recovery Time, Enhanced Performance

Finnish Olympic Ski Team members supplementing colostrum confirm its athletic benefits. Blood creatine-kinase levels were measured over a seven-day period of heavy training. Creatine-kinase is a critically important muscle cell enzyme that acts as a marker for muscle-cell damage. When creatine-kinase levels rise in the blood, there probably has been muscle-cell damage. Compared to ski team members who drank placebos, the athletes who drank a colostrum beverage showed one-half the blood creatine-kinase levels after four days. The individuals in the colostrum supplementation group also reported that they felt better and felt that their performance was improving. The researchers theorize that IGF-I in colostrum could encourage muscle cells to repair themselves more quickly after stress from intense exercise. (Anderson)

"Colostrum is also believed to benefit athletes by enhancing efficiency of amino acid and carbohydrate fuel uptake by the intestines. IGF-I and other factors 'seal' the gut from ulceration, which would reduce uptake efficiency if left unchecked."

Dr. Edmund Burke, Associate Professor of Biology at the University of Colorado, Colorado Springs.

Bovine Colostrum Increase IGF-I in Athletes During Strength and Speed Training

Researchers examined the effects of IGF-1 levels during strength and speed training on athletes supplementing bovine colostrum. Post-training increases were noticed for serum IGF-I in the colostrum treatment and especially in the colostrum treatment compared with the placebo. It appears that a bovine colostrum supplement increases serum IGF-I concentrations in athletes during strength and speed training. (Mero)

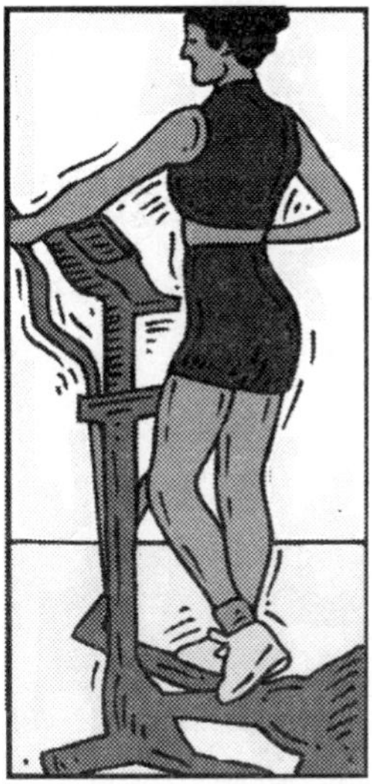

Colostrum and Weight Loss

Increasing levels of IGF-1 is also associated with weight loss as this and other growth factors found in colostrum help the body better utilize the food (especially glucose) you eat. Burning more glucose meaning less is stored and converted to fat.

IGF-1 levels decline as we grow older and also reduced by a lack of exercise, environmental toxins, stress and poor dietary habits. Supplemental colostrum can help restore IGF-1 levels and enhance metabolism, growth of lean muscle tissue and fat burning.

Many people report that their appetite is better balanced when taking colostrum on a regular basis - that they experience less food cravings, and also experience loss of body fat.

TOPICAL USE FOR COLOSTRUM & LACTOFERRIN

It is not surprising that colostrum and lactoferrin are also available in topical application products such as creams. There is not yet much published research on this mode of application, but the potential for benefits definitely exists.

There are many reports that colostrum taken internally is beneficial for skin conditions such as hives and eczema. This, of course, makes perfect sense as these conditions are often allergy related. Anti-inflammatory properties and regulatory factors in colostrum and lactoferrin could be very beneficial.

Tryptase is found in high levels in mast cells in individuals with psoriasis (Harvima), eczema and dermatitis. (Welle, Jarvikallio) Because lactoferrin is known to have an inhibitory effect against tryptase, it is possible that either oral or topical applications would be very beneficial.

Antibiotic and antiviral properties make colostrum and lactoferrin an excellent treatment for various wounds, infections (possibly acne), etc. Epithelial growth factors can help speed healing while anti-inflammatory factors help reduce swelling.

We know that topical applications from colostrum liquid, lozenges or making a paste out of powder and a small amount of water are highly beneficial for periodontal problems.

HOW TO CHOOSE A COLOSTRUM-LACTOFERRIN DIETARY SUPPLEMENT

It is easy to get confused when examining the marketing literature produced by so many companies selling colostrum. Colostrum marketing has been covered in numerous trade and consumer journals and television programs. The following information will be useful to separate fact from fiction and to obtain the best quality product that ultimately lead to the best results for you and your family.

Quality, purity, efficacy, delivery system and price are all important factors in choosing any dietary supplement. The following are the major points you want to consider when selecting a colostrum/lactoferrin supplement:

1. Quality and potency of colostrum and lactoferrin

2. Delivery system

3. Reputation of manufacture

Quality and Potency

Because colostrum and lactoferrin are bioactive, the quality can vary widely from providers. This causes the selection process to be more difficult. To manufacture colostrum, tremendous care must be used in the collection, purification, processing and storage. Colostrum's efficacy is contingent upon the following:

Selection Guide

Collection

True colostrum is obtained in the first milking 3-6 hours after partration. Subsequent milkings contain transitional milk which if blended with the first milking, compromise the delicate balance of immuno-factors in the colostrum. Refer back to the chart on page 46 see how quickly the composition changes after the birth of the calf.

In 1913 the USDH defined colostrum as the milk collected in the first six milkings after partration. This definition was created to prevent colostrum and transitional milk from being sold as milk for human consumption - not to define true colostrum to be used for human immune enhancement–which was unheard of almost 90 years ago.

What this means is that some "so-called colostrum" on the market is not colostrum at all, but actually a whey protein concentrate (WPC). Whey protein concentrate has a very different composition than true colostrum. Only a small amount of true excellent quality colostrum is required to activate an immune system response in the body. Much larger quantities are required from WPC. At 4-16 grams per day, quantities of IGF-1 may be high enough to have some beneficial effect.

After the colostrum is collected it should be frozen and transferred to a processing facility where the fluid is dried under conditions that do not alter or destroy any of its many special components.

- Source of the dairy herd
- Practices of the dairy farmer
- Collection time (optimal: 3-6 hours after delivery)
- Storage and handling of the raw colostrum

Purification

All colostrum raw materials must be tested to be certified free of pathogenic microorganisms. Products should be coded with a lot number that corresponds to laboratory test results.

- Pasteurization techniques
- Whether or not the pasteurized colostrum is modified by removing any:

  lactose
  fat
  casein
  or other component

Processing

Temperatures used to process colostrum should not be above 105 degrees F. in order to preserve its special immune components. At 106 degrees F., enzymes breakdown.

- Spray drying or freeze-drying
- Storage of the dried colostrum
- Processing into liquid, lozenges, capsules or left in powder form

Storage

Some colostrum products may require refrigeration to maintain freshness and optimal shelf life.

- Care in handling and storage by the manufacturer and retailer

Source of the Dairy Herd

Seek a source of colostrum that is in the same geographic location that you currently live in. In other words, if you live in Europe obtain European colostrum. In Asia obtain Asian colostrum. If you live in the United States, obtain U.S. colostrum. The reason is that "local" colostrum is more likely to offer better protection against "local" strains of infectious microorganisms.

Healthy Cattle

Colostrum should come from disease-free herds, in other words - healthy cattle. In the US, they should be Grade A dairy cattle. Dairy cattle, as a general rule, are typically healthier in smaller, closely supervised herds. An average herd size of fifty or so cattle in a family farm are more closely watched, cared for and supervised than a herd of thousands or more. Why? Simple logic. When a farm family makes their living from fifty mature dairy cattle, each cow has a name, a history, and is personally cared for twice a day by the family.

In large herds, employees are hired to care for the animals and the employee's paycheck comes whether or not the herd is carefully watched over or not. It becomes big business and the personal touch...and care are no longer important.

Drug-Free Cattle

Colostrum from cattle raised without exposure to antibiotics, pesticides, and hormones is preferred. These drugs stress and disrupt the normal homeostatic balance in the body.

Antibiotics: The United States produces over 50 million tons of antibiotics annually. Half of these are used for export and the other 25 million tons are given to animals. Most veterinarians use standard antibiotics. U.S. dairy farmers are much more conscious of the fact that whatever they put into their herd will in turn come out in the milk they drink.

Pesticides: Pesticides are widely used in numerous countries in the world. Regardless of the geographic location of the dairy herds, independent assays should be performed on each lot of colostrum to prove safety. If levels are below the standards set for safety, daily use of colostrum will not pose a health threat. Of course, the smallest amount of quality colostrum will yield the least amount of toxins.

It is very difficult to find anything that is 100% pesticide free as residues can be detected in the soil from pesticide use from many decades ago. Feed grown in these soils may contain minute traces of residue even through the farming practice today may be truly "100% organic." Be wary of those who claim "100% pesticide free" - it is not likely unless they brought it in from the moon!

Hormones: Hormones are of two major types: growth and milk production hormones.

Growth hormones are given to young animals in the beef, pork and poultry industries to increase the amount of meat per animal. These hormones are rarely, if ever, given to the animals in a dairy herd.

Milk production hormones cannot be given to a pregnant dairy cow. If the pregnant cow is given milk hormones, she will abort the calf and therefore not produce colostrum. True colostrum is produced by the mother cow prior to giving birth and by definition cannot contain milk production hormones.

Delivery System

Colostrum and lactoferrin products are available as powders in capsules, tablets, chewables, lozenges, as a food additive and in various formulas. Colostrum is also available as a pure liquid, without spray-drying. Creams for topical use containing colostrum and lactoferrin are also available.

Scientific studies with the greatest benefit to the test groups are achieved with the oral delivery of high quality colostrum. Oral delivery means absorption in the mouth, such as sublingually (under the tongue) or slowly dissolving a lozenge. Swallowing hard pressed caplets or capsules is not a true mucosal delivery.

Your delivery decision should also be based upon its intended end use. If you only want to treat the mouth and gums such as in the case of an abcess or periodontal disease, a liquid or powder applied directly to the affect area is likely to be your best choice, although lozenges would work as well. If you are looking to supplement your infants' bottle, then you need a liquid. If you want to treat systemic conditions such as lupus, diabetes, arthritis, asthma, etc., then you need a good mucosal delivery system such as a lozenge.

Reputation of Manufacture

Beware of manufacturers who cut colostrum with whey protein, which has lower levels of immunoglobulins and other important factors. The manufacturer's independent certifications should show the following:

	Colostrum	Whey
Lactose concentration	Very low	Yes
Lactalbumin (a potentially allergenic protein)	None	Yes
IGF-1 content	High	Low
Lactoferrin	High	Low
Immunoglobulins	High	Low
Glycoproteins	High	Low

Be Wary Of False Advertising

Marketing colostrum has become a big business. If you try a certain brand of colostrum and it does not work, don't give up on colostrum. Instead try a different brand, a different form of delivery or both. Remember that many colostrum studies are performed by delivering the colostrum directly into the oral cavity. Capsule delivery of colostrum is likely to not have the same result.

Selection Guide

Some of the false advertising surrounding colostrum includes the following:

1. *Colostrum is the milk-like fluid produced by all female mammals in the first 24 to 36 hours directly after giving birth. It lasts until the onset of lactation, which occurs within 36 to 72 hours post-partum.* **False.** True colostrum is only attained in the first milking after giving birth. After 24 hours, the colostrum is less than one-forth the quality it should be. This would then require a suggested use of more than four times the amount. The sooner it is collected after birth (preferably 3 to 6 hours), the more efficacious it will be.

2. *You can obtain raw colostrum from a dairy farmer.* **False.** The USDA prohibits the sale of raw, unpasteurized colostrum for human use.

3. *If colostrum is frozen, it becomes insoluble in water.* **False**. If colostrum is soluble in water as a liquid, it cannot be rendered insoluble merely by freezing and then thawing. In fact, when colostrum is frozen after harvesting, it will retain its bioactivity longer and will resist the chemical changes that eventually will occur.

4. *Lozenges and tablets are processed using high heat and therefore are ineffective.* **False**. Experienced manufacturers know that cold-pressed lozenges and tablets are not made with high heat. Lozenges and tablets are the preferred method of taking colostrum, so encapsulators generate unfavorable press to make their product more attractive.

5. *Liquid colostrum is not as good as capsules.* **False.** For the same reasons above.

6. *Colostrum should be de-fatted.* **False.** Many of the immuno-factors found in colostrum are contained in the fat. Also, the de-fatting process degrades the colostrum even further.

7. *Colostrum should be de-lactosed.* **False.** Every time colostrum is further processed or an element removed, the colostrum is compromised.

8. *Colostrum is safe for lactose-intolerant individuals.* **Generally false.** The greater the amount of time between birth and collection the greater the lactose content so it depends on the quality of the colostrum. Over 77 mg. lactose will invoke a response in lactose intolerant individuals.

9. *You must take 2 to 4 grams of colostrum daily to receive benefits.* **False.** Just 125 mg. of high quality colostrum taken orally will produce an immune system response.

10. *There is not a good source of colostrum in the United States.* **False.** The United States has several good or excellent providers of colostrum. Also keep in mind that "local" colostrum is preferable.

These are just a few of the false advertising techniques used by unscrupulous manufacturers to promote their product. Read, analyze, ask and try the product. If it doesn't work, try another manufacturer and another form of delivery.

BIBLIOGRAPHY

Aabakken. Lam.: short term effect of bovine colostrum in patients with throat angina. A placebo controlled study. Statistical Report No. 309, Vuramed, Norway. Norges Apatekares tidsskritt, 98 nr 22. April 1990.

Acosta-Altaxuirano. c. et al. 1987. Antlamoebic properties of human colostrum. Adv. Exp. Med. Biol. 216B:1347-52.

Adamik B: Wlaszczyk A d.actoferiin--ita role in defense against infection and Immunotropic properties, Katedra I Elinika Anesteziologli I Inlensywnej Terapli Akademli Medyeniej we Wroclawiu. Postepy Hig Med Dosw 1996;50(1):33-41:

Adamik B; Zimecki M; Wlaszczyk A;et al; Lactoferrin effects on the in vitro immune response in critically ill patients. Dept. of Anesthesiology and Intensive Therapy, U. Medical School, Wroclaw, Poland. Arch Immunol Ther Exp (Warsz) 1998; 46(3): 169-76.

Adamik B; Wlaszczyk A; Lactoferrin--its role in defense against infection and immunotropic properties, Katedra i Klinika Anestezjologii i Intensywnej Terapii Akademii Medycznej we Wroclawiu. Postepy Hig Med Dosw 1996;50(1):33-41.

Adeyemi EO: Campos LB: Lolzou S; et al; Plasma dactoferrin and neutrophil elastase in rheumatoid arthritis and systemic lupus erythematosus Dept of Medicine. Royal Postgraduate Medical School, Hammeramith Hospital, London. Br J Rheumatol 1990 Feb:2911):15-20.

Alugupalli KR; Kalfas S; Inhibitory effect of lactoferrin on the adhesion of Actinobacillus actinomycetemcomitans and Prevotella intermedia to fibroblasts and epithelial cells. Dept of Oral Microbiology, Malmo General Hospital, Lund University, Sweden. APMIS 1995 Feb; 103(2): 154-60.

Amini HR; Ascencio F; Ruiz-Bustos E; Romero MJ; Wadstrom T; Cryptic domains of a 60 kDa heat shock protein of Helicobacter pylori bound to bovine lactoferrin. Department of Medical Microbiology, U of Lund, Sweden. FEMS Immunol Med Microbiol 1996 Dec 31;16(3-4):247-55.

Anderson, 0:; Running Research News. pp 11. January-February, 1994.

Arao S; Matsuura S; Nonomura M; Miki K; Kabasawa K Nakanishi H: Measurement of urinary lactoferrin as a marker of urinary tract infection. Planning and Development Division, Iatron Laboratories, Inc., 1-11-4, Higashikanda, Chiyoda-ku, Tokyo, Japan. J Clin Microbiol 1999 Mar; 37(3):553-7.

Atlinson JC; Yeh C; Oppenhelm FG: et al; Elevation of sallvaiy antimicrobial proteins following HIV- I infection. Clinical Investigations and Patient Care Branch, National Institute of Dental Research, Bethesda, Maiyland. J Acquir Immune Defic Syndr 1990:3(l):4d-8.

Baldwin, Tom. et alp: Elevation of intracedullar free calcium levels In HEp-2 cells infected with enteropathogenic Eseherichia coll. Infection and immunity. (May 199) p. 1599-1604.

Ballard, J.F.. Cl ad.; The Relationship Between the Insulin Content and Inhibitory Effects of Bovine Codostrum on Protein Breakdown in Cultored Cells. Journal of Cellular Physiology (1982) Vol.110,249-254.

Ballard FJ; Nield MK Frands GL Knowles sE; Regulation of Intracellular protein degradation by insulin and growth factors. Acta Blod Med Ger 1981:40(10-11): 1293-300.

Bauxurucker CR Blum JW; Effects of dietary reeomkinant human Insulin-like growth factor-I on concentrations of honnones and growth factees in the blood of newborn calves. J Exxloalnod 1994 Jan. 140(l):15-21.

Bayard BL James MA, Hyperimmune bovine colostnim inefficacious as multiple sclerosis therapy in double-blind study. Department of Food and Nutiltion, University of Wlseonslnstout. Menomonie. J Am Diet Assoc 1987 0ct87(d0): 1388-90.

Baynes RD; Bezwoda WR; Mansoor N; Neutrophil lactoferrin content in viral infections. Am J Clin Pathol 1988 Feb;89(2):225-8.

Ben-Aryeh H, et al. Oral health and salivary composition in diabetic patients. J Diabetes Complications. 1993 Jan-Mar;7(1):57-62.

Bereket A; Lang CH; Wilson TA; Alterations in the growth hormone-insulin-like growth factor axis in insulin dependent diabetes mellitus. Horm Metab Res 1999 Feb-Mar;31(2-3):172-81.

Bertotto A Castellucci G; RadIclOrbi M; Bartolucci M: Vaccaro R, CD4O ligand expression on the surface of colostral T cells. Department of Paedlatrics. Perugla Universlty Medical School. Italy. Arch Dis Child Fetal Neonatal Ed 1996 Mar. 74(21:F135-6.

Bessler H: Straussberg R Hart J: NoW I: Sirota L; Human codostnrm stimulates cytodine production. Hematology and Immunology Research Laboratory, Golda Medical Center, Hashan,n Hospital. Petah-Tiqva. Israel. Biod Neonate 1996:69(6):376-82.

Bezault J; Ilhimani R, Wiprovnick J; Furmanaki P: Human lactoferrln Inhibits growth of solid tumors and development of experimental metastases in mice. New York University, Department of Biology. New York 10003. Cancer Res 1994 May 1,54(91:2310-2.

Bitman J: Hamosh M; Hamosh P: Lutes V; Neville MC; Seacat J; Wood DL; Milk composition and volume during the Onset of lactation in a diabetic mother. Am J Chin Nutr 1989 Dec;50(6): 1364-9.

Bitzan MM; Gold BD; Philpott DJ; et al; Inhibition of Helicobacter pylori and Helicobacter mustelae binding to lipid receptors by bovine colostrum. J Infect Dis 1998 Apr;177(4):955-61.

Bouda, J.. et ad.; Vitamins A and Carotene Metabolism in Cows and their Calves Fed From Buckets. ACTA Vet. Brno. (1980) Vol.49(1-21.45-52.

Bouda. J., et ad.; Vitamins E and C in the Blood Plasma of Cows and their Calves Fed lmm Buckets. ACTA Vet. Bnio. (1980) Vol.49(1-2). 53-58.

Brsmdtzaeq, Per-, The Secretory Immune System of Lactating Human Mammary Gland Compared with other Exoezine Organs. Annals of N.Y. Academy of Science (1983) Vol 409, 353-378.

Bramdtaaeg. P. Annals of the N.Y. Academy of sclerceoo (1983) Vol.409353-378.

Brennan FM, et al. Detection of interleukin 8 biological activity in synovial fluids from patients with rheumatoid arthritis and production of interleukin 8 mRNA by isolated synovial cells. Eur J Immunol. 1990 Sep;20(9):2141-4.

Brock JH; Ismail M: Sanchez L; Interaction of lactoferrln with mononuclear and colon carcinoma cells. University Department of Immunology, Western Infirmary. Glasgow, Scotland. United Kingdom. Mv Exp Med Biol 1994; 357:157-69.

Brock, J. (1995). Lactoferrin: a multifunctional immunoregulatory protein? Immunology Today. 16,9: 417-419.

Brown DL; Kane CD; Chernausek SD; Greenhalgh DG; Differential expression and localization of insulin-like growth factors I and II in cutaneous wounds of diabetic and nondiabetic mice. Am J Pathol 1997 Sep;151(3):715-24.

Buescher ES: The effects of colostrum or neutrophil function: decreased defornability with increased cytoskeletom-assoclated actir. Adv Exp Med Biol 1991:310:131-6.

Bucacher ES; Medlheran SM: Antioxidant properties of human colostrum. Department of Pedlatiles, University of Texas Medical School, Houston 77030. Pedlair Res 1988 Jul:24(1l:14-9.

Buescher ES: The effects of colostrum on neutrophil function: decreased deformability with increased cytoskeletor-associated actir. Mv Exp Med Biod 1991:310:131-6.

Buescher ES: Meldheran SM: Frenck RW: Further characterization of human codostrad antioxidants: identification of an ascorbate-like element as an antioxidant component and demonstmtior of antioxidant heterogeneity. Pedlair Res 1989 Mar,25(3):266-70.

Bueseher. ES. and Meliheran, S.M. 1988. Antloxidant properties of human colostrum. Pedlat. Res. 24:14-19.

Buhler C; Hammon H; et al; Small intestinal morphology in eight-day-old calves fed colostrum for different durations or only milk replacer and treated with long-R3-insulin-like growth factor I and growth hormone. J Anim Sci 1998 Mar;76(3):758-65.

Burke, Edmund. Colostrum as an athletic enhancer and help for AIDS, Nutrition Science News, May 1996. 30-32.

Butte NF: Wong WW; Fiorotto M; Smith EO: Garza C Influence of early feeding mode on body composition of infants. USDA/ARS Children' Nutrition Research Center. Baylor Coliege of Medicine. Houston. Tex.. USA. Biol Neonate 1995:67(61:414-24.

Cameron CM; Kostyo JL, Adamaflo NA; et al; The acute effects of growlln hormone or amino acid transport and protein synthesIs are due to its Insullr-like action. Ann Arbor 48109-0622. Endocrinology 1988 Feb; 122(21:471-4.

Carlson SE. Arachidonic acid status of human infants: influence of gestational age at birth and diets with very long chain n-3 and n-6 fatty acids. J Nutr 1996 Apr;126(4 Suppl):1092S-8S.

Chase, CCL.. et al. 1995. mt effects of oralantiblotic therapies on immune function and productivity. Proc. Am. Assoc. Swine Pract. 26:111-14.

Christensen, Knud. et ad.;: Colostrum treatmert of HIV infected patients with oral pseudomembranous candida infection. European Conference on Clinical Aspects of HIV Infection. Brussels, December 1987.

Close, M. J., Howlett, A. R. Roskelley, C. D. Desprez, P. Y., et al; Division of Life Sciences, Berkeley National Laboratory, University of California, Berkeley, CA October 30, 1997.

Cockburn, F;, Neonatal brain and dietary lipids, Archieves of Disease in Childhood, 1994, 70 F1-F2.

Cortizo AM; Lee PD; Cedola NV; Jasper H; Gagliardino JJ; Relationship between non-enzymatic glycosylation and changes in serum insulin-like growth factor-1 (IGF-1) and IGF-binding protein-3 levels in patients with type 2 diabetes mellitus. Acta Diabetol 1998 Jul;35(2):85-90.

Cregar L; Elrod KC; Putnam D; Moore WR; Neutrophil myeloperoxidase is a potent and selective inhibitor of mast cell tryptase. Departments of Biochemistry and Enzymology, Axys Pharmaceuticals, Inc., South San Francisco, California, Arch Biochem Biophys 1999 Jun 1;366(1):125-30.

Crime Thnes, Vol 2, No. 1, 1986. Mother's Milk increases IQ, reduces neurological problems" The Wacker Foundation, Dept. 132. 1106 North Gflbert Road, Suite 2, Mesa, AZ 85203.

Da Dalt 5: Moncada A Priori N, Valesini G: Pivetti-Pemi P: The lactoferrln tear test in the diagnosis of SJogren's syndrome. Institute of Ophthalmology, University of Roma La Sapienza, Italy. Eur J Ophthalmol 1996 Jul-Sep:6(3):284-6.

Damiens E; El Yazidi I; et al; Role of heparan sulphate proteoglycans in the regulation of humanlactoferrin binding and activity in the MDA-MB-231 breast cancer cell line. Eur J Cell Biol 1998 Dec;77(4):344-51.

Damiens E; Mazurier J; el Yazidi I; Masson M Duthille I; Spik G; Boilly-Marer Y; Effects of human lactoferrin on NK cell cytotoxicity against haematopoietic and epithelial tumour cells. Biochim Biophys Acta 1998 Apr 24;1402(3):277-87.

Dax-wish: Compaxitive Study of Breat Milk of Mothers Deliverylng Preterm and Term Infants- Protein, Fat. and Lactose. Nabnmg. Vol. 33, No. 3 (1989): p. 249.

Defer MC: Dugas B: Picard 0: Damais C: Impairment of clrculating lactoferrin in HIV-1 infection. U313 INSERM, Centre de Recherche des Cordeliers, Paris, France. Cell Mol Biol (Nolsy-le-grand) 1995 May;41(3):417-2159.

Dhaenens L; Szczebara F; Van Nieuwenhuyse S; Husson MO; Comparison of iron uptake in different Helicobacter species. Laboratoire de bacteriologie-hygiene, faculte de medecine Henri- Warembourg, Lille, France. Res Microbiol 1999 Sep;150(7):475-81.

Dohm GL; Elton CW; Raju MS; Mooney ND; et al; IGF-I--stimulated glucose transport in human skeletal muscle and IGF-I resistance in obesity and NIDDM. Diabetes 1990 Sep;39(9):1028-32.

Dial EJ; Hall LR; Serna H; Romero JJ; Fox JG; Lichtenberger LM; Antibiotic properties of bovine lactoferrin on Helicobacter pylori. Department of Integrative Biology, The University of Texas-Houston Medical School. Dig Dis Sci 1998 Dec;43(12):2750-6.

Di Biase N; Napoli A; Caiola S; Buongiorno AM; et al; IGF-1 levels in diabetic pregnant women and their infants. Ann Ist Super Sanita 1997;33(3):379-82.

Dunger DB; Acerini CL; IGF-I and diabetes in adolescence. Diabetes Metab 1998 Apr;24(2):101-7.

Di Poi E, et allL-6 and some natural inhibitors of chronic human inflammation in RA and SLE. Clin Exp Rheumatol. 1999 Jul-Aug;17(4):513.

Ebina T: Sate A Umezu K, Am H: Ishida N: Seki H: Tsukamoto T: 'dYeatment of multiple sclerosis with anti-measles cow codostrum. Med Microbiol Immunol (Berd) 1984:173(2):87-93.

Ebina, T., et al.; Prevention of rotavlrus infection with cow colostrum containing antibody against human rotavlrus. The Lancet. 1983; 29:1029-30.

Ebina T: Ohta M: Kanamaru Y: Yamamoto-Osumi Y: Baba K: Passive immunizations of suckling mice and infants with bovine colostrum containing antibodies to human rotavirus. J Med VIrol 1992 Oct;38(2):117-23.

Ebina T: Sato A Umezu K Ishida N: Ohyama 5: Olzumi A Alkawa K Kataglri 5: Katsushima N: Imal A et ad: Prevention of rotavlrus infection by oral administration of cow codostrum containing antihumanrotavlrus antibody. Med Microbiol Immunod (Berl) 1985:174(4): 177-85.

Elrod KC; Moore WR; Abraham WM; Tanaka RD; Lactoferrin, a potent tryptase inhibitor, abolishes late-phase airway responses in allergic sheep. Arris

Pharmaceutical Corporation, South San Francisco, California. Am J Respir Crit Care Med 1997 Aug;156(2 Pt 1):375-81.

Enestrom S; Bengtsson A; Frodin TDermal IgG deposits and increase of mast cells in patients with fibromyalgia—relevant findings or epiphenomena? Scand J Rheumatol 1997;26(4):308-13.

Falk P; Roth KA; Boren T; Westblom TU; et al: An in vitro adherence assay reveals that Helicobacter pylori exhibits cell lineage-specific tropism in the human gastric epithelium. Proc Natl Acad Sci U SA; 1993 Mar 1;90(5):2035-9.

Fergusson, DM, Beautrais, AL, Silva, PA, Breast-feeding and cognitive development in the first seven years of life. Soc Sci. Med 1982, Vol 16, pp 1705-1708.

Fleener, Scott, Journal of Dairy Science, Vol. 63, Nov. 1980.

Francis, Geofty, Upton, Faye, et al.: Insulln-like growth factors 1 and 2 in bovine colostrum. Biochem J. 1988. 251: 95-103.

Goke B; Fehmann HC; Insulin and insulin-like growth factor-I: their role as risk factors in the development of diabetic cardiovascular disease. Diabetes Res Clin Pract 1996 Feb;30 Suppl:93-106.

Goldman, A and R. Goldhlum: "Human Milk: Imunologic-Nutirltonal Relationship" Micronutrients and Immune Functions, Annals of the New York Academy of Science, Vol. 587(1990) pg 238-243.

Grazioso CF: Buescher ES: Inhibition of neutrophil function by human milk. Cell Immunol 1996 Mar 15:168(21:125-32.

Greenberg PD: Cello JP: Treatment of severe dian'hea caused by Cxypto-sporidium parvum with oral bovine immunoglobulin concentrate in patients with AIDS. J Acquir Immune Defic Syndr Hum Retrovirol 1996 Dec 1:13(41:348-54.

Groenink J; Walgreen-Weterings E; et al; Cationic amphipathic peptides, derived from bovine and human lactoferrin, with antimicrobial activity against oral pathogens. FEMS Microbiol Lett 1999 Oct 15;179(2):217-22.

Grosvenor CE: Plcciano MF: Baumrucker CR Hormones and growth factors In milk Pennsylvania State Universlty, University Park 16802. Endocr Rev 1993 Dec: 14(61:710-28.

Gulve EA, Dice JF: Regulation of protein synthesis and degradation in L8 myotubes. Effects of serum, insulln and insulin-like growth factors. Harvard Medical School, Boston, Blochem J 1989 Jun 1:260(21:377-87.

Hader N; Rimon D; ey al; Altered interleukin-2 secretion in patients with primary fibromyalgia syndrome. Department of Internal Medicine B, Carmel Medical Center, Haifa, Israel. Arthritis Rheum 1991 Jul;34(7):866-72.

Hadorn U, et al. Delaying colostrum intake by one day has important effects on metabolic traits and on gastrointestinal and metabolic hormones in neonatal calves. J Nutr. 1997 Oct;127(10):2011-23.

Hadsell DL: Baumrucker CR Kenslnger RS Effecis of elevated blood Insulin-like growth factor-I (IGF-l) concenlmtion upon IGF-l in bovine mammary secretions during the rolostrum phase. J Endocrlnol 1993 May; 137(21:223-30.

Hanson LA; Mattsby-Baltzer I; Engberg I; Roseanu A; et al; Anti-inflammatory capacities of human milk: lactoferrin and secretory IgA inhibit endotoxin-induced cytokine release. Dept. of Clinical Immunology, U of Goteborg, Sweden. Adv Exp Med Biol 1995;371A:669-72.

Hanson, et al: "Mucosal Immunity" Annals of N.Y. Academy of Science, (1983) Vol 409. 15.

Harmsen MC: Swart PJ: de Bethune MP: et al.: Antiviral effects of plasma and milk proteins: lactoferrin showspotert activity against both human immunodeficiency virus and human cytomegalovirus replication in vim. J Infect Dia 1995 Aug: 172(21:380-8.

Harper, J.M.M., Soar, J.B., and Buttery. J.P.: "Changes in protein metabolism of ovine primary muscle cultores on treatment of grwoth hornone. insulln. insulin-like growth factor I or epidermad growth factor.: J Endocrinology 1987, 112: 87-96.

Harvima IT; Haapanen L; Ackermann L; Naukkarinen A; Harvima RJ; Horsmanheimo MDecreased chymase activity is associated with increased levels of protease inhibitors in mast cells of psoriatic lesions. Department of Dermatology, Kuopio University Hospital, Finland. Acta Derm Venereol 1999 Mar;79(2):98-104.

Hasegawa K; Motsuchi W; Tanaka S; Inhibition with lactoferrin of in vitro infection with human herpes virus. Jpn J Med Sci Biol 1994 Apr;47(2):73-85.

Heinz-Erian P; Achmuller M; et al; Vitamin C concentrations in maternal plasma, amniotic fluid, umbilical cord blood, the plasma of newborn infants, colostrum and transitory and mature breast milk. Padiatr Padol 1987;22(2):163-78.

Hennlngs, J.. et al. 1993. Inimunocoropromlse In gnotobiotic pigs induced h verotoxin-producing Escherichla colt (0111 NM). Infect. Immun. 61:23048.

Hernanz W; Valenzuela A; Quijada J; et al: ;Lymphocyte subpopulations in patients with primary fibromyalgia. J Rheumatol 1994 Nov;21(11):2122-4.

Herrera-Esparza R; Barbosa-Cisneros O; Villalobos- Hurtado R; Avalos-Diaz E; Renal expression of IL-6 and TNF-alpha genes in lupus nephritis. Lupus 1998;7(3):154-8.

Ho. P.C.. Lawton. John. W.M: "Human Codostral Cells: Phagocytosis and Killing of E. Coli and C. Albicans" Infection and immunity (1978) Vol 13, 1433.

Hooton JW: Pabst HF: Spady DW: Paetkau V: Human codosinim contains an activity that inhibits the production of IL-2. Department of Biochemistry, Walter MacKenzie Center, University of Alberta, Edmonton, Canada. Clin Exp Immunol 1991 Dec:86(3):520-4.

Huppertz HI; Rutkowski S; Busch DH; Lissner R; et al; Bovine colostrum ameliorates diarrhea in infection with diarrheagenic Escherichia coli, shiga toxin-producing E. Coli, and E. coli expressing intiminand hemolysin. J Pediatr Gastroenterol Nutr 1999 Oct;29(4):452-6.'

Hurdey WL: Hegarty HM: Melzder JT In vim inhibition of mammaly cell growth by lactoferrin: a comparative study. Life Sci 1994:55(241:1955-63.

Huxley, Dj.. et al. 1995. Evidence supporting the mechanism of enteric protection provided the colostrad wheyed supplements. Proc. Am. Assoc. Bovine Prdct. 27:1938.

Ishiguro Y; Mucosal proinflammatory cytokine production correlates with endoscopic activity of ulcerative colitis. J Gastroenterol 1999 Feb;34(1):66-74.

Itoh Y; Igarashi T; Tatsuma N; et al; Autoimmune fatigue syndrome and fibromyalgia syndrome. Nippon Ika Daigaku Zasshi 1999 Aug;66(4):239-44.

Jara LJ; Lavalle C; Fraga A; et al; Prolactin, immunoregulation, and autoimmune diseases. Semin Arthritis Rheum 1991 Apr;20(5):273-84.

Jarvikallio A; Naukkarinen A; Harvima IT; et al:Quantitative analysis of tryptase- and chymase-containing mast cells in atopic dermatitis and nummular eczema. Br J Dermatol 1997 Jun;136(6):871-7.

Jones BM; Kwok CC; Kung AW; Effect of radioactive iodine therapy on cytokine production in Graves' disease: transient increases in interleukin-4 (IL-4), IL-6, IL-10, and tumor necrosis factor-alpha, with longer term increases in interferon- gamma production. J Clin Endocrinol Metab 1999 Nov;84(11):4106-10.

Juto, P.: Human Milk Stimulates B-Cell Function. Archives of Diseases in Childhood. Vol 60, no 7(1985) pg 610-613.

Kajikawa M; Ohta T; Takase M; et al; Lactoferrin inhibits cholesterol accumulation in macrophages mediated by acetylated or oxidized low-density lipoproteins. Biochim Biophys Acta 1994 Jun 23;1213(1):82-90.

Kalfas S; Andersson M; Edwardsson S; Forsgren A; Naidu AS; Human lactoferrin binding to Porphyromonas gingivalis, Prevotella intermedia and Prevotella melaninogenica. Oral Microbiol Immunol 1991 Dec;6(6):350-5.

Kim. K. et ad.: "In Vitro and In Vivo Neutrallzing Activity of Human Colostrum and Milk Against Purified Toxins A and B of Clostridlum Difficle. J of Infectious DIseases (1984) Vol 150(1) 57-61,

Knutton. Stuart. et ad.: Adhesion of enteropathogenic Escherichia coli to human intestinal enterocytes and cultored human intestinal mucosa. Infection and immunity, Jan 1987. 69-77.

Koenig HL, Schumacher M, Ferzaz B. Thi AN: et al: Progesterone synthesis and myedin formation by Schwann cells. Laboratolre Neurobiodogie du Developpement. Universlte Bordeaux I, Talence. France. Science 1995 Jun 9:268(5216): 1500-3.

Kohl, S.. et ad: "Human Colostral Cytotoxicity: 1. Antibody Dependent Cellular Cytoxdty Against Herpes Simplex VIral-Infected Cells Mediated by Codostesl Cells" Journal of Clinical Laboratory immunology (1978) Vol. 1, 221-224.

Korhonen H; Syvaoja EL; et al: Bactericidal effect of bovine normal and immune serum, colostrum and milk against Helicobacter pylori. Valio Research & Development Centre, Helsinki, Finland. J Appl Bacteriol 1995 Jun;78(6):655-62.

Kuwata H; Yip TT; Tomita M; Hutchens TW; Direct evidence of the generation in human stomach of an antimicrobial peptide domain (lactoferricin) from ingested lactoferrin. Department of Food Science and Technology,University of California, Davis Biochi Biophys Acta 1998 Dec8; 1429(1):129-41.

Laine P; Kaartinen M; Penttila A; Panula P; Paavonen T; Kovanen P; Association between myocardial infarction and the mast cells in the adventitia of the infarct-related coronary artery. Wihuri Research Institute, Helsinki, Finland. Circulation 1999 Jan 26;99(3):361-9.

Lacka B; Grzeszczak W; Genetic aspects of diabetic retinopathy. Wiad Lek 1998;51 Suppl 2:24-9.

Lassus, A,: Colosinim Treatment of aphthous ulcers on the oral mucosa. A placedbo-eontmlled study. Dept of Deinniatodogy. U of Helslnid, Finland. International conference of antimicrobic activity of non-antibloties. Copenhagen. Denmark. 1990.

Lee, CS., et ad, "'Local immunity in the mammary gland'" Veterninary Immunology and immunopatlnyodogy, 32 (1992)1-11.

Lee SS: Lawton JW: Chan CE: Li CS: Kwan Th: Chau EF: Antilactofenin antibody in systemic lupus erythematosus. Medical A. Unit. Queen Elizabeth Hospital. Kowloon, Hong Kong. Br J Rheumatol 1992 Oct.31(l0):669-73.

Leszek J; Inglot AD; Janusz M; et al; Colostrinin: a proline-rich polypeptide (PRP) complex isolated from ovine colostrum for treatment of Alzheimer's disease. A double-blind, placebo-controlled study. Psychiatric Unit, Univ. Medical School, Wroclaw, Poland. Arch Immunol Ther Exp (Warsz) 1999;47(6):377-85.

Lindlahr, H. Philosophy of Natural Therapeutics," LindlahrPublishing Co, Chicago, Ill, 1919)

Lin HH: Kao JH: Hsu HY: et al: Absence of infection in breast-fed infants born to hepatitis C virus-infected mothers J Pedlatr 1995 Api-, 126(4): 589-91.

Lipsitch M; Bergstrom CT; Levin BR; Department of Biology, Emory University, and Department of Epidemiology, Harvard School of Public Health, Proc Natl Acad Sci U S A 2000 Feb 15;97(4):1938-1943.

Li YM; Glycation ligand binding motif in lactoferrin. Implications in diabetic infection. Adv Exp Med Biol 1998;443:57-63.

Li YM; Tan AX; Vlassara H; Antibacterial activity of lysozyme and lactoferrin is inhibited by binding of advanced glycation-modified proteins to a conserved motif. Nat Med 1995 Oct;1(10):1057-6.

Lissner R; Schmidit H; Karch H; A standard immunoglobulin preparation produced from bovine colostra shows antibody reactivity and neutralization activity against Shiga- like toxins and EHEC-hemolysin of Escherichia coli O157:H7. Biotest Pharma GmbH, Dreieich, Germany. Infection 1996 Sep-Oct;24(5):378-83.

Lonnerdal, B; Iyer, S; Lactoferrin: Molecular Structure and Biological Function, Annu Rev. Nutrition, 1995: 13: 93-110.

Lu M: Yao F: Guo A; A study on two gut hormones in breast milki Research Unit of Pediatrics. Xu zhou Medical College. Chung Hun Pu Cham Ko Tsa Chlh 1995 Oct;30(d0):554-6.

Lu XS: Delfi-alasy JF: Grangeot-Keros L Rannou MT PIlot J Rapid and constant detection of HIV antibody response in saliva of HIV-infected patients: selective distribution of anti-HIV activity in the IgG Isotype. Clamart France. Res VimI 1994 Nov-Dec: 145(61:369-77.

Lupia E; Elliot SJ; Lenz O; Zheng F; Hattori M; Striker GE; Striker LJ; IGF-1 decreases collagen degradation in diabetic NOD mesangial cells: implications for diabetic nephropathy. University of Miami School of Medicine, Florida. Diabetes 1999 Aug;48(8):1638-44.

Machnicki M; Zimecki M; Zagulski T Lactoferrin regulates the release of tumour necrosis factor alpha and interleukin 6 in vivo. Laboratory of Immunobiology, Polish Academy of Sciences, Wroclaw. Int J Exp Pathol 1993 Oct;74(5):433-9.

Maimone D; Guazzi GC; Annunziata P IL-6 detection in multiple sclerosis brain. Institute of Neurological Sciences, University of Siena, Italy. J Neurol Sci 1997 Feb 27;146(1):59-65.

Majumdar. Anis A et ad "Protective Properteis of Antichodera Antibodies in Human Colostrum," Infection and immunology. Vol 36, No 36. no.3(1982) pp 962-965.

Manev V; Maneva A; Sirakov L; Effect of lactoferrin on the phagocytic activity of polymorphonuclear leucocytes isolated from blood of patients with autoimmune diseases and Staphylococcus aureus allergy. Sofia, Bulgaria. Adv Exp Med Biol 1998;443:321-30.

Mann, D; Romm,-E; Migliorini,-M. (1994). Delineation of the glycosaminoglycan-binding site in the human inflammatory response protein lactoferrin. J.Biol.Chem. 269,38: 23661-23667.

Manning, A. "The evolution of infections", USA TODAY, 09-30-1997, pp. 04D.

Marchetti M; Pisani S; Antonini G; Valenti P; Seganti L; Orsi N; Metal complexes of bovine lactoferrin inhibit in vitro replication of herpes simplex virus type 1 and 2. Institute of Microbiology, University of Rome La Sapienza, Italy. Biometals 1998 Apr;11(2):89-94.

Markusse HM: van Haexingen W: Swaak AJ: Hogeweg M: de Jong PT Tear fluid analysis in primary Sjogren's syndrome. Clin Exp Rheumatol. 1993 Mar-Apr,1 1(21:175-8.

Marone G; de Crescenzo G; et al; Immunological modulation of human cardiac mast cells. Divisione di Immunologia Clinica e Allergologia, Universita di Napoli Federico II, Italy. Neurochem Res 1999 Sep;24(9):1195-202.

Martinez-Gomis J; Fernandez-Solanas A; et al; Effects of topical application of free and liposome-encapsulated lactoferrin and lactoperoxidase on oral microbiota and dental caries in rats. Arch Oral Biol 1999 Nov;44(11):901-6.

Mattsby-Baltzer I; Roseanu A; Motas C; Elverfors J; et al; Lactoferrin or a fragment thereof inhibits the endotoxin-induced interleukin-6 response in human monocytic cells. Department of Clinical Bacteriology, University of Goteborg, Sweden. Pediatr Res 1996 Aug;40(2):257-62.

Matsuda, T. et al; Il-6/BSF2 in Normal and Abnormal Regultion of Immune Responses, Annals of the New York Academy of Sciences, 1989, Vol: 557, NYAS, NY, 466-476.

McClane SJ; Rombeau JLCytokines and inflammatory bowel disease: a review. Hospital of the University of Pennsylvania, Philadelphia JPEN J Parenter Enteral Nutr 1999 Sep-Oct;23(5 Suppl):S20-4.

Mero A; Miikkulainen H; Riski J; Pakkanen R; Aalto J; Takala T; Effects of bovine colostrum supplementation on serum IGF-I, IgG, hormone, and saliva IgA during training. University of Jyvaskyla, 40351 Jyvaskyla, Finland. J Appl Physiol 1997 Oct;83(4):1144-51.

Miyauchi H; Hashimoto S; Nakajima M; et al; Bovine lactoferrin stimulates the phagocytic activity of human neutrophils: identification of its active domain.Japan.Cell Immunol 1998 Jul 10;187(1):34-7.

Moddoveanu, Zina, et al: Antibacterial Properties of Milk: IgA Peroxidase-Lactoferrir Interactions. Annals of N.Y. Academny of Science (1983) Vol 409.848-850.

Moldofsky H; Sleep, neuroimmune and neuroendocrine functions in fibromyalgia and chronic fatigue syndrome. Adv Neuroimmunol 1995;5(1):39-56.

Molnar I, et al.; High circulating IL-6 level in Graves' ophthalmopathy. Autoimmunity. 1997;25(2):91-6.

Moniuszko T; Rutkowski R; Chyrek-Borowska S; Production of selected cytokines by monocytes (IL-1 beta, IL-6) and lymphocytes (IL-2, IL-4) in peripheral blood of patients with nonallergic bronchial asthma treated with Broncho-Vaxom. Pneumonol Alergol Pol 1995;63 Suppl 2:66-70.

Murphey DK: Buescher ES: Human colosirum has anti-inflammatory activity in a rat subcutaneous air pouch model of inflammatton. Pedlatr Res 1993 Aiig:34(2):208-12. Newberne. P.M., Young. V.R, Naturc (March 23. 1973).

Nakao K; Imoto I; Ikemura N; Shibata T; et al; Relation of lactoferrin levels in gastric mucosa with Helicobacter pylori infection and with the degree of gastric inflammation. Am J Gastroenterol 1997 Jun;92 (6):1005-11.

Nakao K; Imoto I; Gabazza EC; Yamauchi K; et al; Gastric juice levels of lactoferrin and Helicobacter pylori infection. Scand J Gastroenterol 1997 Jun;32(6):530-4.

Naudin J; Mege JL; Azorin JM; Dassa D; Elevated circulating levels of IL-6 in schizophrenia. Service du Pr Azorin, CHU Sainte-Marguerite, Marseille, France. Schizophr Res 1996 Jul 5;20(3):269-73.

Nawata, Y., et al; Il-6 is the Principal Factor Produced by Synovia of Patients with Rheumatoid Arthritis that induces B-lymphocytes to secrete immunoglobulins. Annals of the New York Academy of Sciences, 1989, Vol: 557, NYAS, NY, 230-238.

Neurath MF; Fuss I; Schurmann G; Pettersson S; Arnold K; Muller-Lobeck H; Strober W; Herfarth C; Buschenfelde KHCytokine gene transcription by NF-kappa B family members in patients with inflammatory bowel disease. Laboratory of Immunology, University of Mainz, Germany. Ann N Y Acad Sci 1998 Nov 17;859:149-59.

Neuringer, M.; Reisbick, S.; Janowsky, J.; The Role of n-3 fatty acids is visual and cognitive development: Current edidence and methods of assesment. The Journal of Pediatrics, 1994, Vol. 125,:5, Part 2 S39-S47.

The New England Journal of Medicine, Intravenous Immune Globulln For the

Prevention of Bacterial Infections in Children wtth Symptomatic Human Immuno Deficiency Virus Infections.(July 11, 1991)325:73-80.

Noda. Kovichi, et al. Transforming Growth Factor Activity in Human Colostrum: Gannoo (1984) Vol.75, 109-112.

Noni, Jill, Pearl Map David DlJohn, Saul Tsiporoo and Carol 0. Tacket: Treatment With Bovine Hyperimmune Colostrum of Cxytosprbdlal Dlanhea in AIDS Patients. AIDS (1990)4:581-584.

Nord J; Ma P; DiJohn D; Tzipori S; Tacket CO; Treatment with bovine hyperimmune colostrum of cryptosporidial diarrhea in AIDS patients. St Vincent's Hospital and Medical Center, NY. AIDS 1990 Jun;4(6):581-4.

Ogra. Pearay. et al.: Annals of New York Acedemy of Science. (1983) Vol. 409.82-92.

Ogra. Pearay. et al.: Colosirum derived Immunity and Maternal Neonatal Interaction. Annals of NY Acedemy of Science (1983) Vol. 409, pp 82-92.

Oldham, G.: Suppression of bovine lymphocyte responses to mitogens following in vivo and in vitro treatment with dexamethasone. Veteminary Immunology and Immunopathyology, 320 (1992)161-177.

Peen E; Johansson A; Engquist M; Skogh T; Hepatic and extrahepatic clearance of circulating human lactoferrin: an experimental study in rat. Department of Medical Microbiology, Faculty of Health Sciences, Linkoping University, Sweden. Eur J Haematol 1998 Sep;61(3):151-9.

Pell, J.M.. and Bates, P.C.: Manipulation of growth and muscle protein metabolism by exogenous insulln-like growth-factor 1 and growth honnone. Acts Paedlair Scand (Supple) 367:161.

Petschow BW; Talbott RD; Batema RP; Ability of lactoferrin to promote the growth of Bifidobacterium spp.in vitro is independent of receptor binding capacity and iron saturation level. J Med Microbio l1999 Jun;48(6):541-9.

Plettenherg A Stoehr A Stellbrink I-U: Albrecht H MeigelW.: A preparation from bovine colostrun in the treatment of HIV-positive patients with chronic diarrhea. Clin Investig 1993 Jam7l(1):42-5.

Pollanen MT; Hakkinen L; Overman DO; Salonen JI; Lactoferrin impedes epithelial cell adhesion in vitro. J Periodontal Res 1998 Jan;33(1):8-16

Prokopiv MM: larosh AA, Effect of colostnim on the enzymatic function of the liver in patients with multiple sclerosisi. Vrach Delo 1988 Apr,(4): 100-2.

Puddu P; Borghi P; Gessani S; et al; Antiviral effect of bovine lactoferrin saturated with metalions on early steps of human immunodeficiency virus type1 infection. Int J Biochem Cell Biol 1998 Sep 30(9):1055-62.

Punzi L, et al. Interrelationship between synovial fluid interleukin (IL)-6, IL-1 beta and disease activity indices in rheumatoid arthritis. Rheumatol Int. 1994;14(2):83-4.

Rice KD; Tanaka RD; Katz BA; Numerof RP; Moore WRInhibitors of tryptase for the treatment of mast cell-mediated diseases. Curr Pharm Des 1998 Oct;4(5):381-96.

Rodriguez-Ortega. Morella. et al,: Membrane glycoproteins of humm polymorphonuclear leukocytes that act as receptors for mannose-specific escherichla coli. Infection and Immunity. April 1987, 968-973.

Rodriguez M; Pavelko KD; McKinney CW; Leibowitz JL Recombinant human IL-6 suppresses demyelination in a viral model of multiple sclerosis. Department of Neurology, Mayo Clinic, Rochester, MN. J Immunol 1994 Oct 15;153(8):3811-21.

Rogler G; Meinel A; Lingauer A; Michl J; Zietz B; Gross V; Lang B; Andus T; Scholmerich J; Palitzsch KD; Glucocorticoid receptors are down-regulated in inflamed colonic mucosa but not in peripheral blood mononuclear cells from patients with inflammatory bowel disease. Eur J Clin Invest 1999 Apr;29(4):330-6.

Rouse. B.T., et al.: Antibody-Dependent Cell Mediated Cytotoxicity in Cows: Comparison of Effector Cell Activity Against Heterologous Erythrocyte and Herpes virus-infected Bovine Target Cells. Infection and immunity (1976) Vol 13. 1433.

Rump JA Arndt K Arnold A Bendick C: Diehteimuller H: Franke M: Heim EB: Jager H: Kampmann B: Kolb P: et ad.: Treatment of diarrhea in human immunodeficiency virus-infected patients with immunoglobulins from bovine codostrum. Clin Investig 1992 Jul:70(71:588-94.

Saha K Dun N: Chopra K Use of human colostrum in the management of chronic infantile diarrhea due to enteropathogenic E. colt infection with associated intestinal parasite infestations and undernutrition. J TropPedlair 1990 Oct:36(51 :247-50.

Saito H; Asakura K; Ogasawara H; et al; Topical antigen provocation increases the number of immunoreactive IL-4- , IL-5- and IL-6-positive cells in the nasal mucosa of patients with perennial allergic rhinitis. Int Arch Allergy Immunol 1997 Sep;114(1):81-5.

Sallh, Y.. LR McDowell, J.F. Hentges. R.M. Mason. C.J. Wilcox: Mineral Content of Milk, Colostrum, and Serum as Affected by Physiological State and Mineral Supplementation. Journal of Dairy Science (1987) Vol.70(3), 608-612.

Samborski W; Lacki JK; Wiktorowicz KE; The lymphocyte phenotype in patients with primary fibromyalgia. Ups J Med Sci 1996;101(3):251-6.

Samnson. R., et ad.: Inununology (1979) Vol. 381 (2), 376-73.

Saniholm. M.. et ad, (1979) Colostral Trypsin-Inhibitor Capacity in Different Animal Species, Acta Veteninaria Scandinavica. Vol. 20. (41.469-476.

Sarker SA; Casswall TH; Mahalanabis D;et al; Successful treatment of rotavirus diarrhea in children with immunoglobulin from immunized bovine colostrum. Pediatr Infect Dis J 1998 Dec;17(12):1149-54.

Schmidt AM, et al. Regulation of human mononuclear phagocyte migration by cell surface-binding proteins for advanced glycation end products. J Clin Invest. 1993 May;91(5):2155-68.

Segev Y; Landau D; et al; Growth hormone receptor antagonism prevents early renal changes in nonobese diabetic mice. J Am Soc Nephrol 1999 Nov;10(11):2374-81.

Shing. Yuen and Elagabrun, Micheal: Purification and characterization of a bovine Colostrumderived growth factor. Molecular Endocrlnolocy 1987, 335.

Siciliano R, et al. Bovine lactoferrin peptidic fragments involved in inhibition of herpes simplex virus type 1 infection. Biochem Biophys Res Commun. 1999 Oct 14;264(1):19-23.

Singleton, P; Sainsbury, D.; Dictionary of Microbiology and Molecular Biology, 2nd ed. 1996. Wiley.

Skotiner, V.: Anabolic and Tilsue Repair Functions of Recombinant Insulin-Like Growth Factors I, Acta Pediatr Scand (SupplI 376:367:63-66, 1990.

Snydennan. Ralph, M.D.: Advances in Rheumatology. Medical Clinics of North America. (Mamth 1986) Vol.70(21,217.

Sporn, MB.. et al. "Polypeptide Transforming Growth Factors Isolated From Bovine Sources and used for Wound Healing in Vivo" Science (1983) Vol 219. 1329-1331.

Staroscik, K.. et al. "Immunologically Active Nonapeptide Fragment of a Proline-Rich Polypeptide from Ovine-Colostrum: Amino And Sequence and lmmuno-regulatoiy Properties" Molecular immunology (1983) Vol. 20(121. 1277-1282.

Stromqvist M; Falk P; Bergstrom S; Hansson L; et al; Human milk kappa-casein and inhibition of Helicobacter pylori adhesion to human gastric mucosa. J Pediatr Gastroenterol Nutr 1995 Oct;21(3):288-96.

Subratty AH; Hooloman NK; Role of circulating inflammatory cytokines in patients during an acute attack of bronchial asthma. Indian J Chest Dis Allied Sci 1998 Jan-Mar;40(1):17-21.

Swaak AJ, et al. Cytokine production (IL-6 and TNF alpha) in whole blood cell cultures ofpatients with systemic lupus erythematosus. Scand J Rheumatol. 1996;25(4):233-8.

Ritchie, and Becker 1994 titis Update on the management of intestinal cryptosporidlosis in AIDS. Ann-Pharmacol. 28:767-78

Rouse. B.T. et at.. 1976. Antibodydependent Cell-mediated cytotoxicity in cows: Comparison of cifector cell activity against heterologous erythroeytes and herpesrus-Infected bovlne target cells. Infect. Immun. 13:1 433A0.

Salvi M, et al. Increased serum concentrations of interleukin-6 (IL-6) and soluble IL-6 receptor in patients with Graves' disease. J Clin Endocrinol Metab. 1996 Aug;81(8):2976-9.

Swart PJ: Kulpers ME: et al; Antiviral effects of milk pmtelns: acylation results in polyanionic compounds with potent activity against human immunodeficiency virus types 1 and 2 in vitro. AIDS Res Hum Retroviruses 1996 Jun 10: 12(9):769-75

Swart PJ: Kulpers ME: et al.: Antiviral effects of milk proteins: acylation results in polyanlonic compounds with potent activity against human immunodeficiency virus types 1 and 2 in vitro. AIDS Res Hum Reimviruses 1996 Jun 10: 12(9):769-75.

Swart, P,J et al. (1996). Antiviral effects of milk proteins: Acylation results in polyanionic compounds with potent activity against human immunodeficiency virus types 1 and 2 in vitro. AIDS-RES-HUM-RETROVIRUSES. 12,9: 769-775.

Swart PJ; Kuipers EM; Smit C; Van Der Strate BW; Harmsen MC; Meijer DK; Lactoferrin. Antiviral activity of lactoferrin. Department of Pharmacology, University of Groningen, The Netherlands. Adv Exp Med Biol 1998;443:205-13.

Tanaka K; Ikeda M; Nozaki A; Kato N; Tsuda H; Saito S; Sekihara H. Lactoferrin inhibits hepatitis C virus viremia in patients with chronic hepatitis C: a pilot study. Third Department of Internal Medicine, Yokohama City University School of Medicine, Yokohama. Jpn J Cancer Res 1999 Apr; 90(4):367-71.

Taylor, B, Wadsorth, J; Breastfeeding and child development at five years Developmental Medicine and Child Neurology, 1984, 26. pg. 73-80.

Tenovuo J; Lumikari M; Soukka T; Salivary lysozyme, lactoferrin and peroxidases: antibacterial effects on cariogenic bacteria and clinical applications in preventive dentistry. Proc Finn Dent Soc 1991;87(2):197-208.

Theodore, Christine. et al.: "Immunologic Aspects of Colostrum and Milk: Development of Antibody Response to Respiratory Syncytial Virus and Bovine Serum Albumin in the Human and Rabbit Mammary Gland" Recent Advances in Mucosal Immunity (1982) (Raven Preas), New York.

Tokuyama H: Tokuyama Y: Bovine colostre transforming growth factor-beta-like peptide that induces growth inhibition and changes in morphology of human osteogenic sarcoma cells (MG63). Cell Biol int Rep 1989 Mar.13(3):251-8.

Thomas, Frank et al.: Increased weight gain, nitrogen retention and muscle protein zynthesis following treaiment of dinbetic rats with IGF-I anddes 1-3 (IGF-I). BlochemJ. 1991,276: 547- 554- 547

Thomas. Frank et a.: Effects of full-length and trunicated insulin-like growth factor-l on nitrogen balance and muscle protein metaholism in nitrogen restrcted rate. J Endocrinology 1991, 128: 97-105.

Toner, M. "Science Watch: Antibiotics' Nemesis: Bacteria that become resistant to the 20th century's wonder drugs are: hardier, longer-lasting adversaries than scientists had suspected." The Atlanta Journal and Constitution; 12-07-1997.

Tritschler, P. HJ, Wolff, S.P., Thioctic (lipoic) acid: a therapeutic metal-chelating antioxidant? Biochem Pharmacol 1995 Jun 29;50(1):123-6.

Tsai WJ: Uu HW: Yen JH: Chen JR Lin SF: Chen TP: Lactoferrin in rheumatoid arthritis and systemic lupus erythematous. Kao Hsiung I Hsueh Ku Hsueh Tsa Chili 1991 Jan: 7(l):22-6.

Tzipori 5: Roberton D: Cooper DA: White L: Chronic cryptosporidlal diarrhea and hyperimmune cow colostrum Idetterd. Lancet 1987 Aug 8:2(8554):344-5.

Tyrell, David,: Breast Feeding and Virus Infection The Immunity of Infant Feeding. (1980) Plenum Press, N.Y.. 55-61.

Ulcova-Gallova Z, et al.; Immunologic factors in human colostrum and milk. Cas Lek Cesk. 1994 May 2;133(9):275-6.

Urban, T. The Oponizing ability in antibodies from some health care products containing bovine colostrum. State Laboratory, State Phannaceutical Company. Stockhoim. Swedish Phannaceutical Asociation, Yearly Congress, 1990.

van Leeuwen MA; Westra J; Limburg PC; van Riel PL; van Rijswijk MH Interleukin-6 in relation to other proinflammatory cytokines, chemotactic activity and neutrophil activation in rheumatoid synovial fluid. Ann Rheum Dis 1995 Jan;54(1):33-8.

Vassilev it: Veleva KV: Natoral polyreactive IgA and 1gM autoantibodles in human colosinim. Seand J immunol 1996 Nov.44(5):535-9.

Viander B: Ala-Uotila 5: Jalkanen NI: Pakkanen R, Viable AC-2. a new adult bovine serum- and codostrum-based supplement for the culture of mammalian cells. Blotechniques 1996 Apr,20(41:702-7.

Von Fellenberg, Fl,: Hoeber, H;: Multiple protease Inhibitors in and Codosinim and in bovine udder tissue and their possible significance. Schwelz. Arch. Tlerheilkd. 1980.122 (31. 159-66.

Vorland LH; Ulvatne H; Andersen J; Haukland H; Rekdal O;et al; Lactoferricin of bovine origin is more active than lactoferricins of human, murine and caprine origin. Scand J Infect Dis 1998;30(5):513-7.

Wada T; Aiba Y; Shimizu K; Takagi A; Miwa T; Koga Y; The therapeutic effect of bovine lactoferrin in the host infected with Helicobacter pylori. Scand J Gastroenterol 1999 Mar;34(3):238-43.

Wads. N. et al.: Neutralizing Activity Against Ckxstridium Difficile Toxins in the Supernatant of Cultured Colostral Cells. Inictious Immnunology (1980) Vol 29.545-550.

Ward, C.G. Bullen, J.J., Rogers, H.J.; Iron and Infection: New Developments and their Implications, Journ of Trauma, Injury, Infection and Critical Care, 1996, Vol 41:2, 356-364.

Wadsteinm J, The use of colosirum immuglobulines against gastrointestinal disorders, mouth infections and cutaneous infections, University of Lond. Sweden (Feb 1991).

Wakabayashi H; Okutomi T; Abe S; Hayasawa H; Tomita M; Yamaguchi Hy, Morinaga Enhanced anti-Candida activity of neutrophils and azole antifungal agents in the presence of lactoferrin-related compounds. Adv Exp Med Bio 11998;443:229-37.

Ward, P.P; Zhou, X; Conneely, O.M. (1996). Cooperative interactions between the amino-and carboxyl- terminal lobes contribute to the unique iron-binding stability of lactoferrin. J. Biol. Chem. 271,22: 12790-12794.

Watanabe T: Nagura H: Watanabe K; et al: The binding of human milk lactoferrin to immunoglobulin A. FEBS Left 1984 Mar 26: 168(2):203-7.

Weldham, RH., et al; Annals of N.Y. Academy of Science., (1983) 409. 510-515.

Welle MM; Olivry T; Grimm S; Suter M; Mast cell density and subtypes in the skin of dogs with atopic dermatitis. J Comp Pathol 1999 Feb;120(2):187-97.

Wester TJ; Fiorotto ML; Klindt J; Burrin DG; Feeding colostrum increases circulating insulin-like growth factor I in newborn pigs independent of endogenous growth hormone secretion. ARS, USDA, Department of Pediatrics, Baylor College of Medicine, Houston, TX. J Anim Sci 1998 Dec;76(12):3003-9.

Wlaszczyk A; Zimecki M; Adamik B; Durek G; Kubler A: Immunological status of patients subjected to cardiac surgery: effect of lactoferrin on proliferation and production of interleukin 6 and tumor necrosis factor alpha by peripheral blood mononuclear cells in vitro. Arch Immunol Ther Exp (Warsz) 1997;45(2-3):201-12.

Wootan, George, "Take Charge of Your Child's Health"" Crown Publishers. Inc. New York (1992) pg 111-135.

Wong WW: Hachey DL: Insull W: Opekun AR, Klein PD: Effect of dietary cholesterol on cholesterol synthesis in breast-fed and formula-fed infants. USDA/ARS Children's Nutrition Research Center, Department of Pediatrics, Baylor College of Medicine, Houston, TX. J Lipid Flea 1993 Aug:34(81:1403-11.

Woywodt A; Ludwig D; et al: Mucosal cytokine expression, cellular markers and adhesion molecules in inflammatory bowel disease. Eur J Gastroenterol Hepatol 1999 Mar;11(3):267-76.

Xu Ri: Development of the newborn Gl tract and is relation to codostrum/milk intake: a review. Department of Zoology, University of Hong Kong, Reprod Fertil Dev 1996:8(11:35-48.

XuY Y; Samaranayake YH; Samaranayake LP; Nikawa H Invitro susceptibility of Candida species to lactoferrin. School of Stomatology, Beijing Medical University, China. Med Mycol 1999 Feb; 37(1):35-41.

Yamauchi K; Wakabayashi H; Hashimoto S; Teraguchi S Hayasawa H; Tomita M.; Effects of orally administered bovine lactoferrin on the immune system of healthy volunteers. Adv Exp Med Biol 1998;443:261-5.

Yavuzyilmaz E; Yumak O; Akdoganli T; et al; The alterations of whole saliva constituents in patients with diabetes mellitus. Aust Dent J 1996 Jun;41(3):193-7.

Ye S: Sun R, Lu 9: The study of growth factors in human colostrmm. Nanjing University.

Yoo YC; Watanabe S; Watanabe R; Hata K; Shimazaki K; et al., Bovine lactoferrin and Lactoferricin inhibit tumor metastasis in mice. Adv Exp Med Biol 1998;443:285-91.

Zimecki M; Spiegel K; Wlaszczyk A; Kubler A; Kruzel ML; Lactoferrin increases the output of neutrophil precursors and attenuates the spontaneous production of TNF-alpha and IL-6 by peripheral blood cells..Arch Immunol Ther Exp (Warsz) 1999;47(2):113-8.

Zimecki M; Wlaszczyk A; Cheneau P; Brunel A; et al; Immunoregulatory effects of a nutritional preparation containing bovine lactoferrin taken orally by healthy individuals. Institute of Immunology and Experimental Therapy, Polish Academy of Sciences, Wroclaw, Poland. Arch Immunol Ther Exp (Warsz) 1998;46(4):231-40.

Zimecki M; Miedzybrodzki R; Szymaniec S Oral treatment of rats with bovine lactoferrin inhibits carrageenan- induced inflammation; correlation with decreased cytokine production. Arch Immunol Ther Exp (Warsz) 1998;46(6):361-5.

Zimecki M; Wlaszczyk A; Zagulski T; Kubler A; Lactoferrin lowers serum interleukin 6 and tumor necrosis factor alpha levels in mice subjected to surgery. Arch Immunol Ther Exp (Warsz) 1998;46(2):97-104.

INDEX

Bordtella 48

ABOUT THE AUTHOR

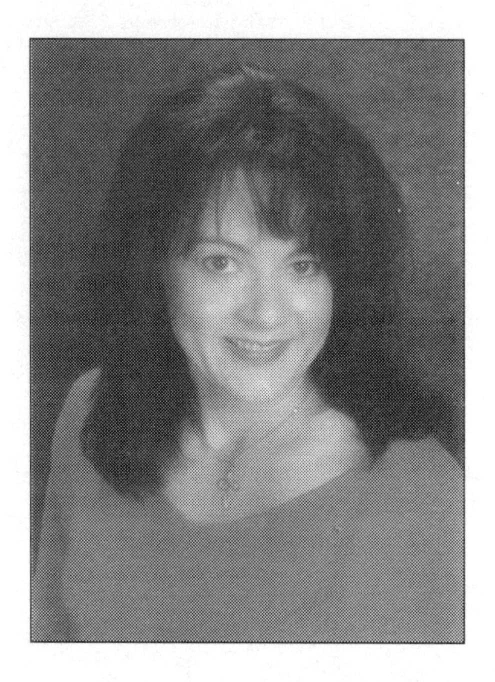

Beth M. Ley, Ph.D., has been a science writer specializing in health and nutrition for over 10 years. She wrote her own undergraduate degree program and graduated in Scientific and Technical Writing from North Dakota State University in 1987 (combination of Zoology and Journalism). Beth has her masters (1997) and doctoral degrees (1999) in Nutrition.

Beth lives in the Minnesota lakes country. She is dedicated to God and to spreading the health message. She enjoys spending time with her Dalmatians, exercises on a regular basis, eats a vegetarian, low-fat diet and takes anti-aging supplements.

Memberships: American Academy of Anti-aging, New York Academy of Sciences, Oxygen Society.

Other Contributors

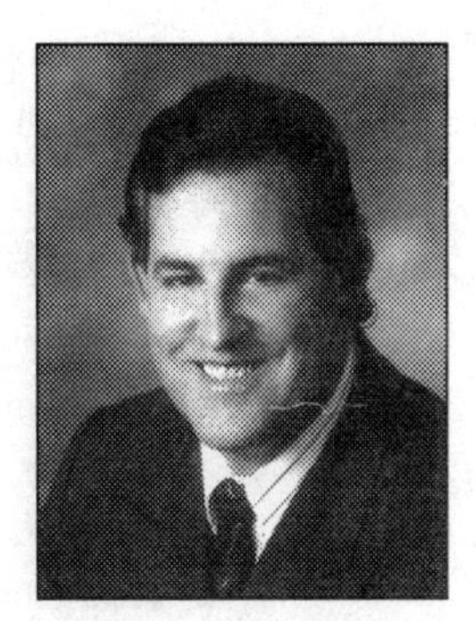

Raymond Lombardi, D.C., N.D., C.C.N., received his Doctorate of Chiropractic from Palmer College of Chiropractic West, in 1991. In 1997 he obtained his certification as a Clinical Nutritionist. In 1998 he received his certifications as a Clinical herbalist and a board certified Naturopathic Physician. He is currently continuing his education through the School of Natural Healing, Salt Lake City, UT.

Dr. Lombardi, author of *Aspirin Alternatives* (BL Publications, 1999) and *Modern Chiropractics (1993)*, has also published a number of articles appearing in *Better Nutrition, Health Keepers,* and *Energy Times* magazinesand is a frequent guest speaker on national radio shows.

Dr. Lombardi presently has an alternative-care holistic practice in Redding, CA.

Kenneth D. Johnson, S.M.D., S.N.D., O.M.D., Ph.D., of San Jose, CA., received a triple major international Ph.D. from Olympian International Sports College in Bratislava, Czechoslovakia in 1989 in international sports medicine, sports nutrition and oriental medicine. Dr. Johnson was also named a fellow in the college with the following titles: Fellowship of Olympian International Sports Medicine College, Fellowship of Olympian International Sports Nutrition College, Fellowship of Olympia International Oriental Medicine College and Fellowship of Olympian International Sports College.

In 1988 Dr. Johnson was asked to serve on the International Olympian Nutrition Committee for the 1988 Olympics Games in Seoul, Korea. Following the 1988 Olympics Dr. Johnson was appointed Director of Sports Nutrition for the Olympian International Sports Federation at the 1992 Olympic Games in Barcelona, Spain.

Recognized internationally as a healer, researcher, author, lecturer and teacher, Dr. Johnson is a highly sought after professionally by schools, associations, health care practitioners, physicians and patients worldwide.

ORDER THESE GREAT BOOKS
FROM BL PUBLICATIONS!

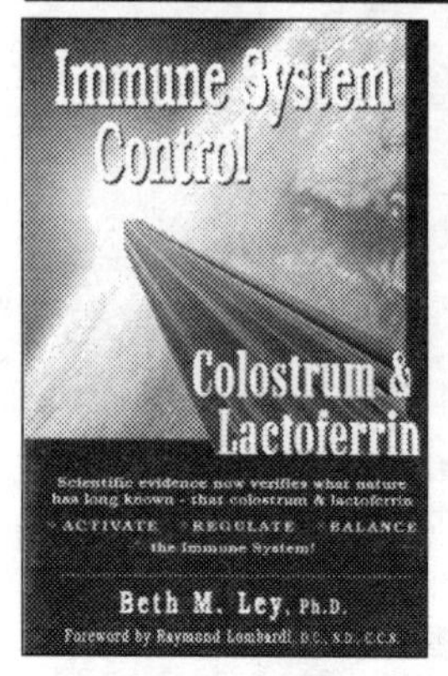

Immune System Control Colostrum & Lactoferrin
Beth M. Ley, Ph.D. 200 pages, $12.95
ISBN 1-890766-11-9
Get the FACTS about colostum and lactoferrin! Featuring a special product selection guide! Fully referenced/Indexed

Marvelous Memory Boosters Beth M. Ley, Ph.D. 2000, 32 pages, $3.95

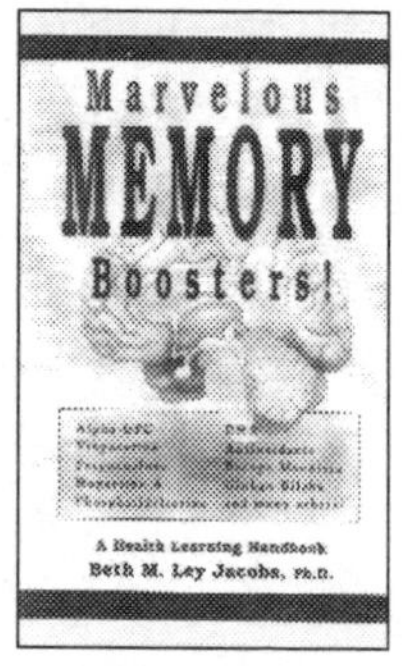

Aging, exposure to brain toxins, nutritional deficiencies & other factors contribute to memory loss & deterioration of other mental capabilities. Certain nutrients & phytochemicals (Alpha GPC, Vinpocetine, Huperzine-A, Pregnenolone, Phospholipids, DHA, Bacopa Monniera, Ginkgo Biloba, etc.) improve short & long term memory, increase mental acuity & concentration, improve learning abilities & mental stamina, reduce fatigue, improve sleep, mood, vision & hearing.

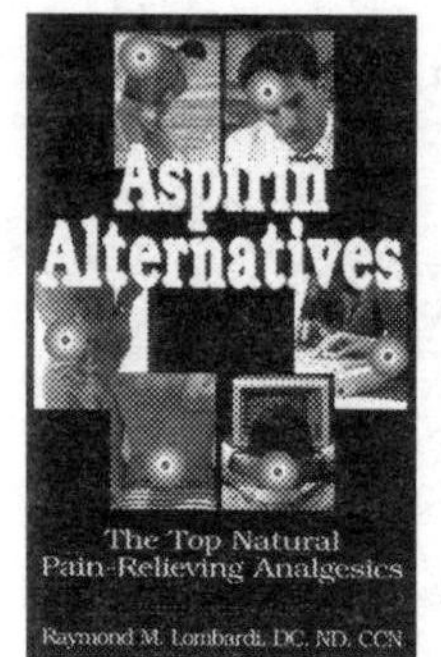

Aspirin Alternatives: The Top Natural Pain-Relieving Analgesics
Raymond Lombardi, D.C., N.D., C.C.N., 1999, 160 pages, $8.95

This book discusses analgesics and natural approaches to pain. Ibuprofen and acetaminophen are used for pain-relief, but like all drugs, there is a risk of side effects and interactions, There are a number of natural alternatives which are equally effective and in many cases may be preferable because they may help treat the underlining problem rather than simply treating a symptom.

Vinpocetine: Boost Your Brain w/ Periwinkle Extract! Beth M. Ley, Ph.D. 2000, 48 pgs. $4.95

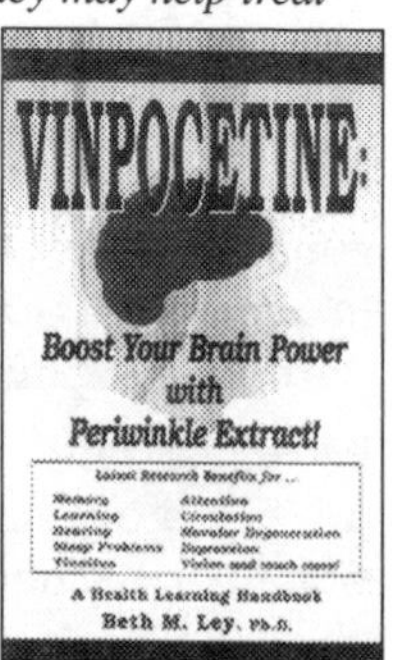

This herbal extract benefits: Memory, attention and concentration, learning, circulation, hearing, insomnia, depression, tinnitus, vision & more! Vinpocetine increases circulation in the brain and increases metabolism in the brain by increasing use of glucose and oxygen. Benefits both the old and young!

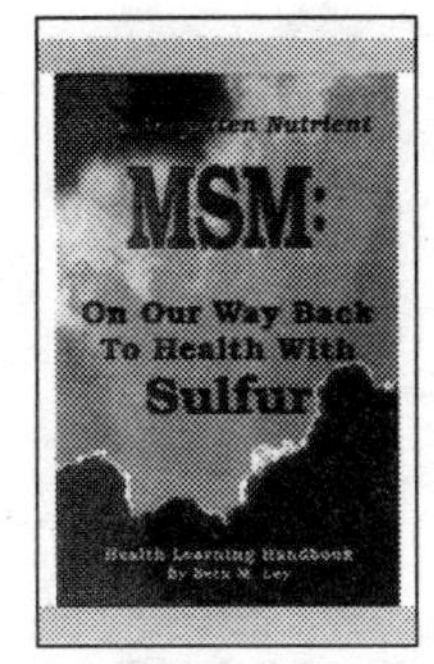

MSM: On Our Way Back To Health With Sulfur

Beth M. Ley, 1998, 40 pages, $3.95

MSM (methyl sulfonyl methane), is a rich source of organic sulfur, important for connective tissue regeneration. Beneficial for arthritis and other joint problems, allergies, asthma, skin problems, TMJ, periodontal conditions, pain relief, and much more! Includes important "How to use" directions.

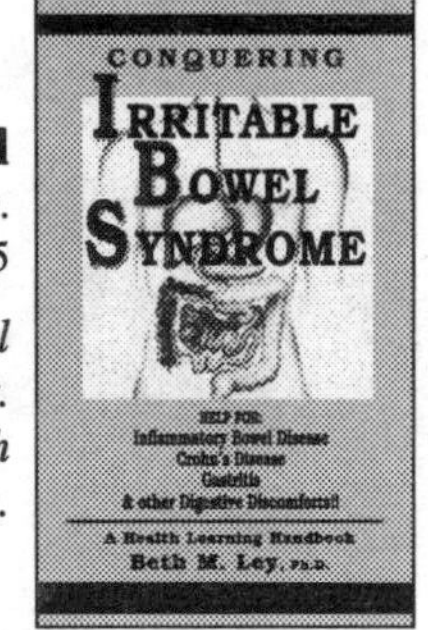

Conquering Irritable Bowel Syndrome!

Beth M. Ley, Ph.D. 2000, 92 pages, $6.95

Irritable bowel is the most common gastrointestinal problem today yet there is no effective medical treatment. Learn how to overcome this painful problem through natural supplements and dietary modifications.

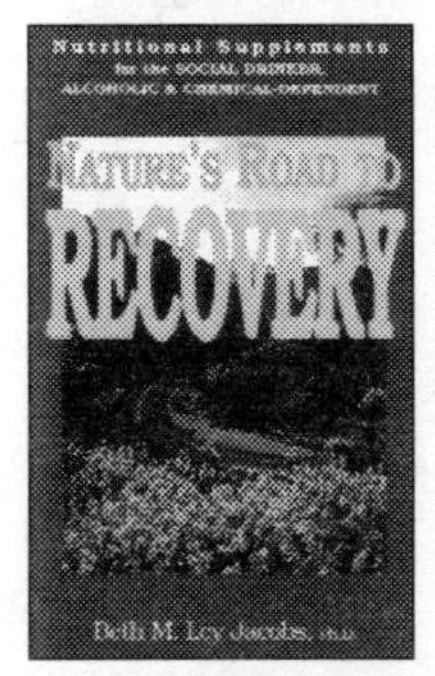

Nature's Road to Recovery: Nutritional Supplements for The Social Drinker, Alcoholic & Chemical-Dependent

Beth M. Ley-Jacobs, Ph.D., 1999, 72 pages, $5.95

Recovery involves much more than abstinence. Cravings, depression, memory loss, liver problems, vascular problems, sexual problems, sleep problems, nutritional deficiencies and common health problems which can benefit from 5-HTP, DHA, phospholipids, St. John's Wort, antioxidants, etc.

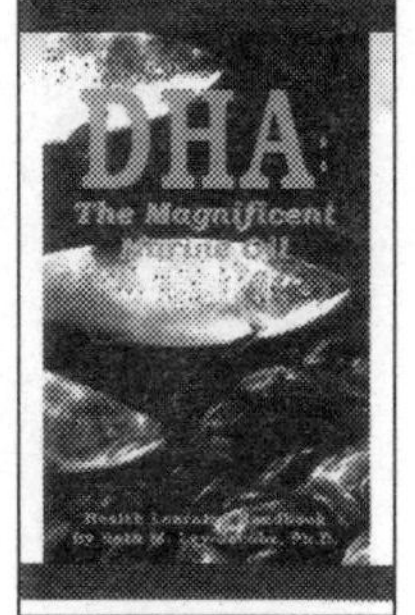

DHA: The Magnificent Marine Oil

Beth M. Ley-Jacobs, Ph.D., 1999, 120 pages, $6.95

Individuals commonly lack this essential Omega-3 fatty acid so important to the brain, vision, and immune system and much more. Memory, depression, ADD, addiction disorders (especially alcoholism), inflammatory disorders, skin problems, schizophrenia, elevated blood lipids, etc., benefit from DHA.

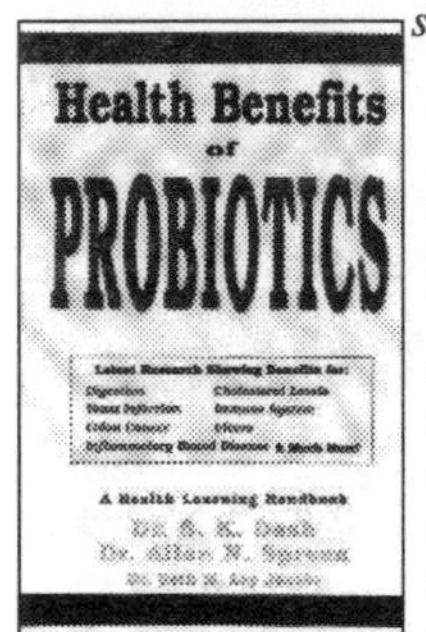

Health Benefits of Probiotics

Dr. S.K. Dash & Dr. Allen Spreen 2000, 56 pages, $4.95

Probiotics aid in the maintenance of the healthy balance of intestinal flora. They improve digestion, cholesterol levels, immunity; Correct digestive disorders, ulcers, inflammatory bowel diseases, lactose intolerance, yeast infections; Help prevent colon cancer; Reduce side effects of antibiotics & more!

Coenzyme Q10: All Around Nutrient for All-Around Health!

Beth M. Ley-Jacobs, Ph.D., 1999, 60 pages, $4.95

CoQ10 is found in every living cell. With age, insufficient levels become more common, putting us at serious risk of illness and disease. Protect and strengthen the cardiovascular system; benefit blood pressure, immunity, fatigue, weight problems, Alzheimer's, Parkinson's and Huntington's Diseases, gum-disease and slow aging.

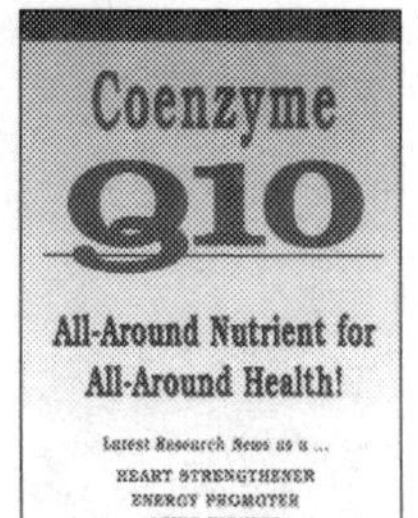

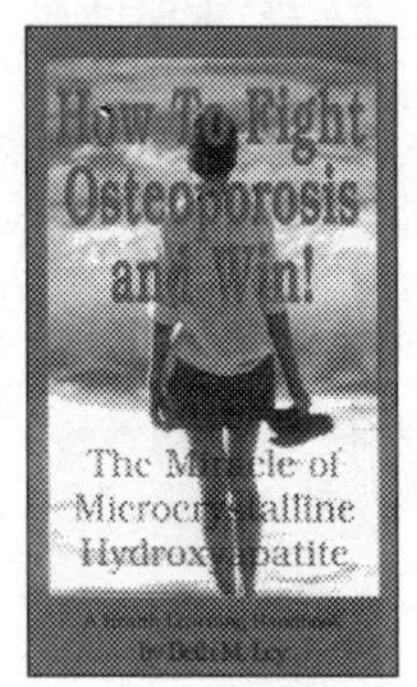

How to Fight Osteoporosis & Win: The Miracle of MCHC

Beth M. Ley, 80 pgs. $6.95

Find out if you are at risk for osteroporosis and what to do to prevent and reverse it. Get the truth about bone loss, calcium, supplements, foods, MCHC & much more! Find out what supplements can help you most!

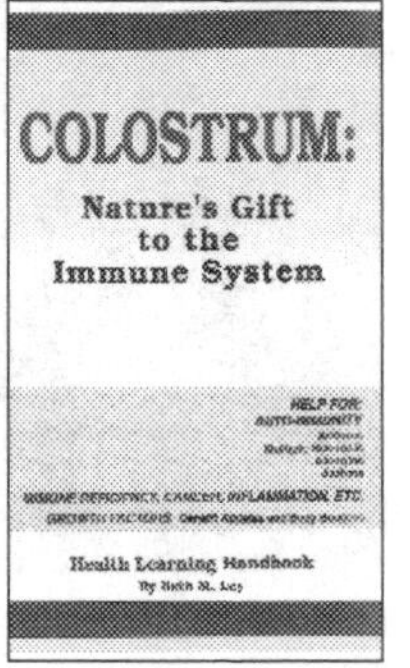

Colostrum: Nature's Gift to The Immune System, Beth M. Ley, 80 pages, $4.95

An earlier edition - Colostrum, "first milk," is rich in immuno-factors such as antibodies, growth factors, lactoferrin, etc., which can boost & support the immune system of everyone!

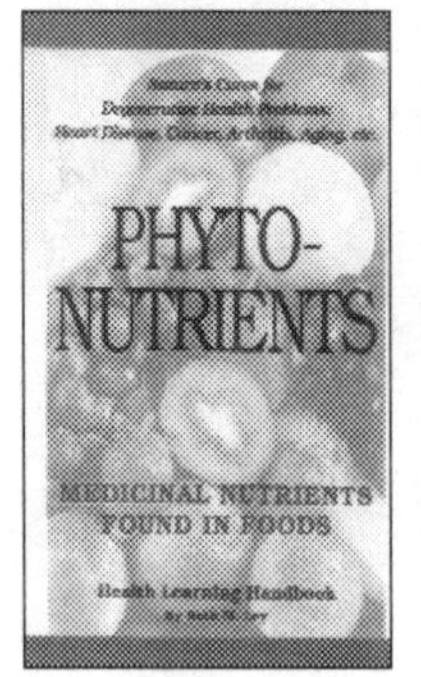

Phyto-Nutrients: Medicinal Nutrients Found in Foods, Beth M. Ley, 40 pgs. $3.95

Learn about special components in our foods which protect our health by fighting off disease & aging! Learn about onions, garlic, flax, bilberry, green tea, red wine, rosemary, cruciferous vegetables, cayenne pepper, ginger, soybeans, avacados, beets, cranberries, sweet potatoes, amaranth, etc.

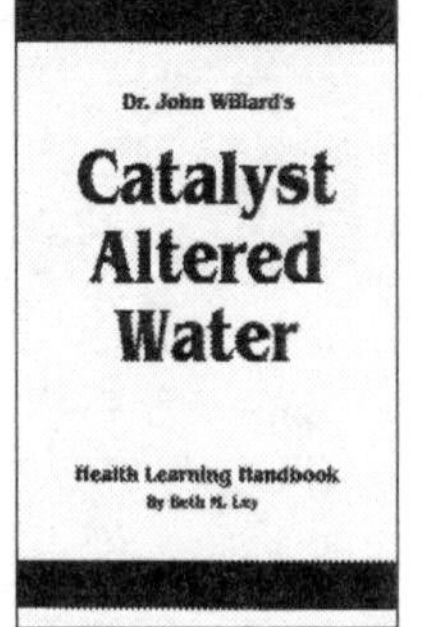

Dr. John Willard's Catalyst Altered Water Beth M. Ley, 80 pgs. $3.95

Learn about the amazing properties of "Willard Water," how to use it for plants, pets, cleaning, drinking & specific health problems ranging from arthritis to burns.